Freedom From Food: An Overview

Welcome to The Waist Away Bible Study! Get ready to meet new friends and get out of bondage to food. We encourage you to go through this process in a small group because accountability is the key to creating the habits for permanent weight loss. You have no special foods to buy, and you are never going to need pre-packaged foods like Nutrisystem® or Jenny Craig® again! You will actually save money because by incorporating fasting you will eat much less food than you were before. Again, we recommend you go through this process in a group, but if you cannot, then consider signing up for coaching at https://chantelrayway.com/get-coaching/.

As you lose weight, we would love to read your testimony/see your before/after pics. Email them to questions@chantelrayway.com or submit them at https://chantelrayway.com/onemealaday/.

This workbook is most effectively used as a companion to both *Fasting to Freedom* and *Waist Away*, which will give you insight into the physical and spiritual benefits and necessity of fasting.

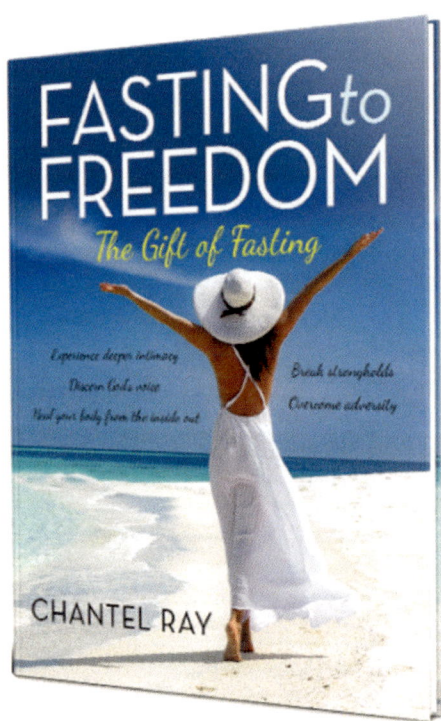
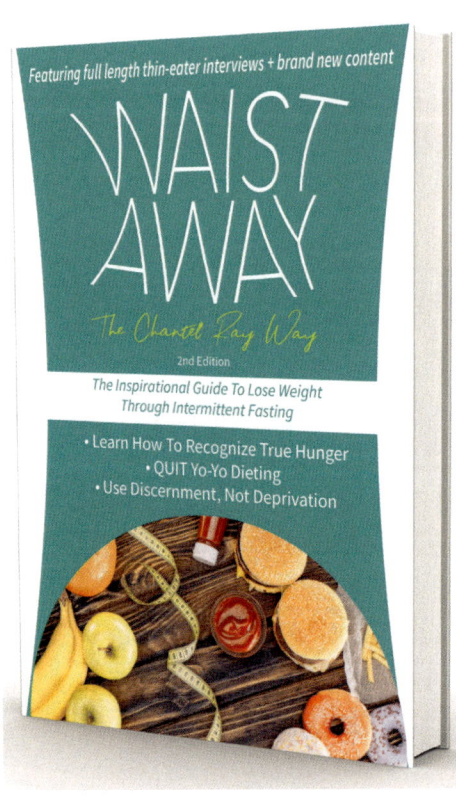

Overview

This process is based on 5 key principles called the FIRES Principles. You will get a quick overview of these, but the two most important principles you will learn are: I: Identify True Hunger and S: Stop Before You're Full. In this course, you will learn that you have true hunger and fake hunger. True hunger is your stomach's desire for fuel. Fake hunger is the desire to eat because of emotional reasons. Come up with your own wording choice to remember the emotions that drive you to eat when you're not truly hungry like: loneliness, sadness, boredom, anxiety, frustration, and happiness. There is nothing wrong with drinking alcohol, shopping, or eating foods you enjoy. The problem comes with overdoing any of these things. **You must learn that the only time you should put food in your mouth is when you're physically hungry not emotionally hungry, or you will never be free from the bondage of food.** We all have some kind of hurt in our lives and for so long, people have used food as a tool to mask that hurt. It will take time to unlearn this, but it is possible.

Do you have to be a Christian to do this program?

No. Whether you believe in God or not, you can do this program! However, this workbook is written from a foundation of faith.

Why Diets Don't Work

The problem with diets is that they force us to focus more on food. They create a big greed problem because instead of addressing the problem of overeating, they actually encourage us to have more food than we need. They justify it by labeling some foods as "good" and others as "bad." Eventually our willpower will fail, we will give into those cravings and end up overeating. Diets put you in a position where you're almost worshiping food because it becomes such a focus. You might be able to lose weight on some of these low-carb, low-calorie, low sugar-diets even if you're overeating, but at some point, you will go back to the foods you really want. This is because you never addressed the main issue: overeating. You never learned to listen to your signs of hunger and fullness. The Bible instructs us to refrain from gluttony. Thin eaters don't focus on food that much. Thin eaters can even forget to eat.

Session 1: Overeating Is a Sin

Weekly Ice Breaker

Peaks and Pits – Think about the past week. What were your Peaks and your Pits?

These can be food/eating-related but don't have to be. Your Peaks should be things that brought you joy, made you feel happy, made you smile, made you feel energized or excited – things you enjoyed and would enjoy doing again. Your Pits should be things that drained your energy, made you upset or angry, made you sad, made you frustrated, or gave you a headache – things you wish you didn't have to repeat again.

Now, write them in the spaces below:

Peaks	Pits

Weekly Game

Find One in Five. Everyone thinks of something unusual about themselves related to food or eating (like an unusual food they've eaten). Then they have five seconds to find one person who has the same thing in common with them. Once they find someone, yell out, "FOUND ONE!" Then do it again, but this time they must find two people, and so on. Whoever finds the most things in common with others wins!

FIRES Activity

Pick a partner and take 3 minutes to list all the emotions/adjectives that come to mind when you think of the following words. Whichever team comes up with the most words that no one else has wins! (Do not read ahead on next page)

❶ Fireplace: (ex: comforting)

❷ Fireworks: (ex: exciting)

❸ House Fire: (ex: devastating)

FIRES Activity Application:

Think about all the words you came up with:

Fireplace: cozy, comforting, family, snuggly, warm, romantic, safe, love

Fireworks: exciting, bright, fun, holiday, family, celebration, joyful, happy, loud

House Fire: devastating, destruction, powerless, nervous, fear, terror, pain, loss

All these emotions/words relate to reasons you overeat. Some people overeat for comfort or when they have family gatherings. Some people overeat on holidays or when they're out having fun. Some people overeat when they feel powerless or when they're sad or scared.

I overeat when I feel powerless. Personal Example: I have 3 web developers on staff, but one day SalesForce, which is the computer system that drives our company, had a glitch, so everything came to a halt at work. Even though I was a math major in college and actually minored in computer programming, this was way beyond my expertise. I felt powerless, so I ate. I also tend to eat when I feel physically weak or sick because I mistakenly think the food will make me feel better.

❶ Which of these emotions is the #1 reason you overeat?

❷ Are there any other emotions we are missing that make people overeat?

THE 5 FIRES PRINCIPLES

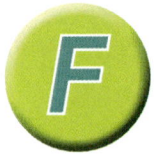

Fast On A Regular Basis

The Lord calls us to fast. He uses the word "when" and not "if" to show that it is expected of us!

Matthew 6:16-18
"When you fast, do not look somber as the hypocrites do, for they disfigure their faces to show others they are fasting. Truly I tell you, they have received their reward in full. But when you fast, put oil on your head and wash your face, so that it will not be obvious to others that you are fasting, but only to your Father, who is unseen; and your Father, who sees what is done in secret, will reward you."

Identify True Hunger

To understand hunger, you have to properly define it. Hunger is the physical need for fuel. It's something that comes in cycles. You're never hungry all the time. Hunger is also something that we often confuse with appetite. Appetite is your mental desire for food. You can have an appetite all the time.

Psalm 63:5
I will be fully satisfied as with the richest of foods; with singing lips my mouth will praise you.

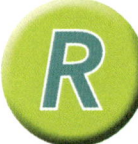

Reduce Sugar

Try to eat 80% real clean foods and 20% whatever you're craving. The question you're going to ask is, "Why not eat clean 100% of the time?" Trying to eat perfectly will cause you to feel deprived and lead to binging.

1 Corinthians 6:19-20
Do you not know that your bodies are temples of the Holy Spirit, who is in you, whom you have received from God? You are not your own; you were bought at a price. Therefore, honor God with your bodies.

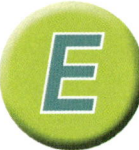

Enjoy Real Food Without Deprivation

You DON'T have forbidden fruits. As soon as something is a forbidden fruit in your mind, you crave it. There is no forbidden fruit in this lifestyle. There is nothing you can't eat. You are re-introducing yourself to food and you are CHOOSING to eat healthful foods most of the time. I eat a little bit of something every day that would be considered "off-limits" on a traditional diet. You just want to remember to rate your foods and only eat what you really want.

Romans 12:1
Therefore, I urge you, brothers and sisters, in view of God's mercy, to offer your bodies as a living sacrifice, holy and pleasing to God—this is your true and proper worship.

Stop Before You're Full

The best thing you can do to help you decide when to stop eating is to eat what you really want. Savoring your food is easier when you're eating only what you really want.

Proverbs 23:2
...and put a knife to your throat if you are given to gluttony.

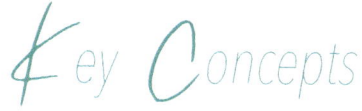

Key Concepts

If your gas tank were full, would you try to put more gas into it?

No!

It would just lead to a mess and damage your car! Why, then, do we put more food into our bodies when we are already full?? Try to think of your body as that full gas tank. Do not put more fuel into it when it is already full!

Application Questions

? When do you refill your car's gas tank? Is it ¼ full? All the way on E? _____

? When do you refill your stomach? Is it ¼ full? All the way on E? _____

You must acknowledge that overeating is a sin.
As long as you're pretending that gluttony is fine, you're never going to repent and turn away from your behavior.

Sin leads to slavery.

Overeating, just like any other sin, can be addictive.

You become a slave to your own habits. It's a vicious cycle because the more you overeat the more you want to overeat.

Because our bodies are temples of the Holy Spirit, there are privileges and responsibilities regarding how we care for ourselves.

1 Corinthians 3:16-17

Don't you know that you yourselves are God's temple and that God's Spirit dwells in your midst? If anyone destroys God's temple, God will destroy that person; for God's temple is sacred, and you together are that temple.

One thing every thin eater reports is that she hates the feeling of overeating. It makes her tired/sluggish/uncomfortable

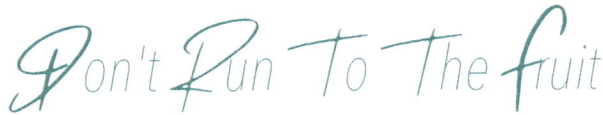

One of the girls in my small group said, "When I'm stressed, I'll run for something healthy like strawberries, so even if I overeat, it's good for me." This is not true! If you run to foods like celery or carrots when you aren't physically hungry, it is a sin because you are still using food for comfort or for reasons other than hunger. You must retrain your body to never overeat, even on foods that you consider "good." The whole point is that you must find something else in place of snacking or eating when you are not physically hungry. For example, if you are on a diet you may decide, "Okay, I am going to have nothing but veggies and lean meats for a week and nothing else." Then you get a call at work and are completely stressed out, and your first reaction is: "I'm stressed; I need to go eat carrots!" Carrots may be healthful, but you have still trained your body to go to food, even though you are not hungry. You must retrain your brain to know that if you aren't physically hungry, you cannot eat or snack, even if it is just a carrot stick. If you eat carrots, broccoli, a kale smoothie, or whatever you choose every time you're stressed, you might end up losing weight because you are reducing your caloric intake, but you still are training your body to run to food anytime you are feeling a negative emotion.

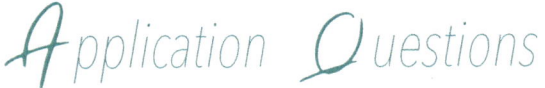

? How often do you overeat?

_____

? Are there certain triggers that make you overeat?

_____

? Do you feel shame after you overeat?

_____

? Watch the video at chantelrayway.com/biblestudy called, "When Do You Stop Eating." At what point do thin eaters stop eating?

_____

Gray Areas

There are areas in the Bible that I believe are gray, meaning Scripture doesn't speak on them specifically. When the Bible neither condemns nor condones certain behaviors, like gambling, people often go back and forth on whether they are permitted or prohibited. Gray areas are those where the Bible gives no direct command, leaving people to use other verses to try to justify their position on the behavior. Here are some common gray areas:

- ○ Getting a nose piercing
- ○ Getting a tattoo
- ○ Dancing
- ○ Wearing a bikini
- ○ Listening to secular music
- ○ Drinking a beer

Application Questions

❓ Which of the above gray areas do you think are permitted? Why?

_____

❓ Can you name any other gray areas in the Bible?

_____

However, I think the Bible is very black and white when it comes to two issues involving eating:

Overeating is prohibited: In the Bible, overeating is referred to as gluttony. Gluttony is the sinful enjoyment of the gift of food; it's eating to the point of greed. There are many verses condemning gluttony.

Proverbs 23:21
For drunkards and gluttons become poor, and drowsiness clothes them in rags.

Proverbs 23:2
...and put a knife to your throat if you are given to gluttony.

Proverbs 28:7
A discerning son heeds instruction, but a companion of gluttons disgraces his father.

1 Corinthians 6:13
You say, "Food for the stomach and the stomach for food,
and God will destroy them both."

Eating when you're not physically hungry is prohibited: If you eat when you're not physically hungry, I believe you're making food an idol because using food for anything other than physical fuel for body, like for emotional reasons, turns it into an idol.

> *An idol is anything that we live for, or that we crave, or that controls us. You can spend your life preoccupied with idols and what they can offer you. If you put anything ahead of God in your life, and it is in direct competition with God, it is an idol. Dieting and food plans can be an idol. Trying to be too thin and obsessing about your body can be an idol.*

There are many Bible verses prohibiting idols:
If you're living a life where you weigh yourself several times a day, you're counting every point, you're counting every calorie that goes into your mouth, or counting every macro or every carb, then most likely you're obsessing to a point that you've made food and dieting your idol.

Application Questions

Exodus 34:17
Do not make any idols.

Leviticus 19:4
Do not turn to idols or make metal gods for yourselves. I am the LORD your God.

1 Samuel 12:21
Do not turn away after useless idols. They can do you no good, nor can they rescue you, because they are useless.

? Can you name any other idols that people worship instead of God?

_____

? Even things that seem positive, like working out, can be idols, if they become your go-to. Can you think of any other positive things that people turn into idols?

_____

Mark 7:18-23

"Are you so dull?" he asked. "Don't you see that nothing that enters a person from the outside can defile them? For it doesn't go into their heart but into their stomach, and then out of the body." (In saying this, Jesus declared all foods clean.)

He went on: "What comes out of a person is what defiles them. For it is from within, out of a person's heart, that evil thoughts come–sexual immorality, theft, murder, adultery, greed, malice, deceit, lewdness, envy, slander, arrogance and folly. All these evils come from inside and defile a person."

Diets try to pretend that some foods are more "spiritual" than others, but the above passage teaches us that's not true. Jesus says food in and of itself isn't spiritual. Note: While I say that, I do believe that there is a lot on the market today that isn't real food, but just chemicals in a package.

The Sneaky Smoothie Story

I want to share a story about my friend, Crystal, who lives down the street. Her husband started making a smoothie every day for breakfast and talked her into having a smoothie every day too. She is a thin eater and never wanted breakfast and never ate till 1 or 2 pm, but her husband convinced her that breakfast was the most important meal of the day, so she started drinking the smoothies too. They had protein powder, banana, spinach, and other fruit and were probably about 400-500 calories. She drank these for about 2-3 months and changed nothing else in her diet. You aren't going to believe it, but she gained 10 lbs! All it took was her drinking this one smoothie that she didn't really want. Here's a thin eater who followed her husband's bad advice, and it caused her to gain 10 lbs. The point is you must always follow your own hunger and fullness cues!

Application Questions

? Do you have a similar story where you ate outside the confines of hunger and fullness because a podcast, friend, etc. told you to, and it made you end up gaining weight?

_____

"Harmless" Lies

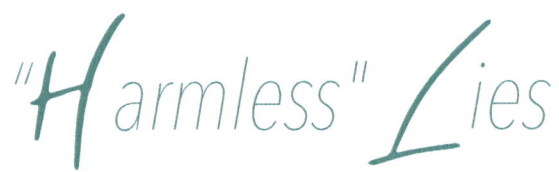

The Devil likes to use lies to try to tempt us. He tries to convince us that there's a legitimate reason we should give into temptation. The more we tell ourselves these lies, the easier it is to convince ourselves that they're true. That's why it's important that we recognize each time we tell ourselves a lie, or believe one that is told to us. Look at these categories of lies. Did you tell yourself any of these lies, or something similar, this week? If so, what did you tell yourself?

☐ **Being Rude Lie:**
Example: "My friend is taking me out for my birthday. It would be rude for me not to eat."

_____

☐ **Time of Day Lie:**
Example: "It's noon; it's time to eat."

_____

☐ **Reward Lie:**
Example: "I've worked so hard all day, and today was so stressful. I need to reward myself and go out for a big meal even though I'm not hungry."

_____

☐ **Clean Your Plate Lie:**
Example: "I hate not to eat everything on my plate because there are starving children in Africa."

_____

☐ **Free Meal Lie:**
Example: "My boss is taking us out for free meal. I already ate lunch, but it's free, so I'll eat again."

_____

☐ **Never Getting This Again Lie:**
Example: "Grandpa is taking us to Ruth's Chris. I'll never get steak this good again, so I better eat it all."

_____

A Meal And A Tasting

As I interviewed more and more thin women I eventually realized there was a pattern to how they ate. Most of them ate a meal and a tasting. That is the formula that works best for me now, as well. I eat 2 times a day: 1 medium to large meal consisting of whatever I want depending on my hunger, and my next meal is just a tasting of about 9 bites. I might eat 3 bites of 3 different things; it's actually more of a snack than a meal.

Food Freedom

- One of the things that really helped me to get to a place where I wasn't making food an idol was finding complete Food Freedom. What I mean by Food Freedom is that instead of obsessing about food and letting it control you, you take control of what you eat so that what goes into your body is what you truly want.

- For a while, I took all gluten and dairy out of my diet and then reintroduced it back in small amounts till my body could process it again. Now I can eat it in small amounts, and I'm fine.

- Before that, I was eating so cleanly that it almost became an idol. I was so obsessed that I had to relearn the idea of Food Freedom.

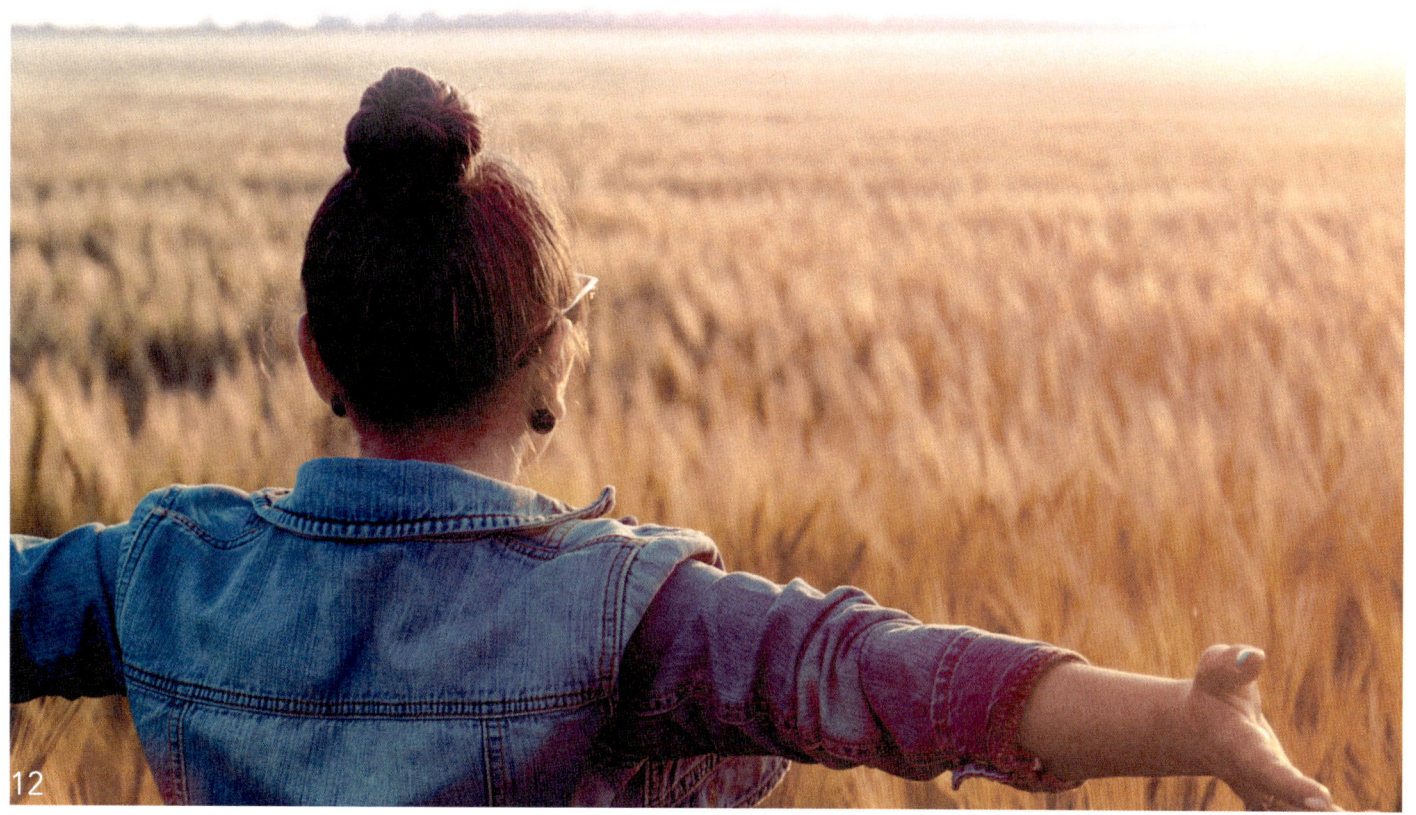

I'd like to clarify a few different sensations that affect the food habits we have. Where are you in terms of balance?

Neurotic Nutrition:
A complete obsession with clean eating and getting all the proper nutrients.

Food Freedom:
You are in control of your choices and aren't thinking about food every second of the day. You aren't obsessed with stringent rules and can eat whatever you want as long as you're truly hungry and stop before you're full.

Being Balanced:
Finding your balance of different food groups that fulfill your nutritional needs and also keep you mentally satiated. For me it's 80% clean foods and 20% whatever I want. For others it's 70/30 and for some it's 60/40. Being balanced is the difference between being educated or obsessed. You should educate yourself about the things that are good for your body but not let it become an obsession or an idol.

Where Does Your Hunger Come from?

Do you know what true hunger feels like? Review these mimics and true hunger, below:

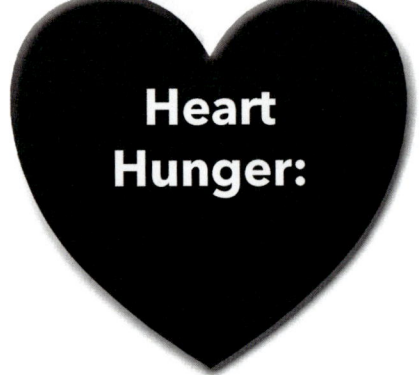

Head Hunger: It is a mindless hunger. You eat because it's there and it looks good, it's impulse: you see a commercial for Taco Bell® and start to crave it, or someone brings Krispy Kreme® doughnuts to work, and they look good, so you eat one even though you aren't hungry.

Heart Hunger: Emotional eating, using food for comfort, companionship, anger, sorrow, anxiety.

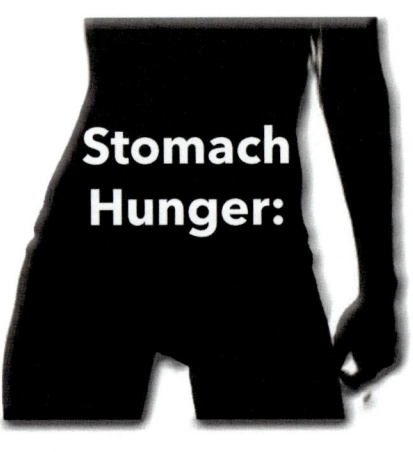

Stomach Hunger: Actual true hunger.

Food can't satisfy heart or head hunger; it can only satisfy true stomach hunger.

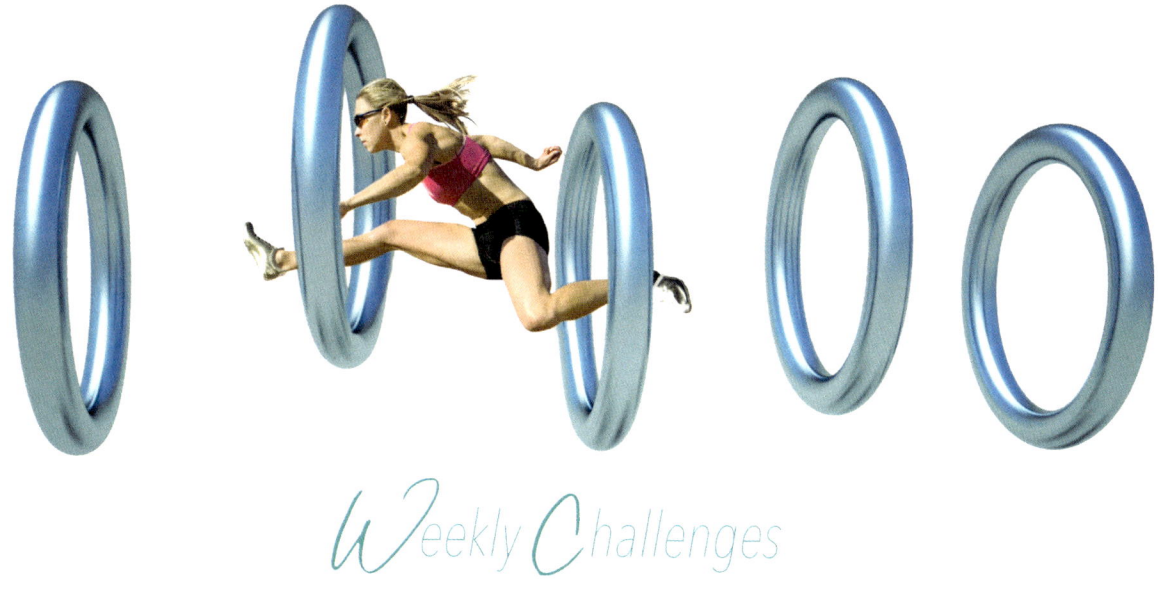

Weekly Challenges

A. **Choose an Accountability Partner:** Overeating isn't something you need to hold in. Tell somebody about it and gain control. Talking about your problem with someone you trust provides support and accountability. You need both of these to be healed of your overeating.

James 5:16
Confess your sins to each other and pray for each other so that you may be healed.

Accountability Partner:

Name: _____

Email: _____

Phone number: _____

B. **Weigh Yourself** on Monday morning, and record your weight. Weigh yourself again on Sunday evening, and record your weight.

_____   _____
Monday Morning Weight   Sunday Night Weight

C. **Use a Journal** to record every time you eat when you're not truly hungry. See if you can find a pattern/ trigger.

D. **Memory Verse:**

Proverbs 23:2
...and put a knife to your throat if you are given to gluttony.

E. Make *THREE* Weekly Commitments:

Here are some examples:

1. Waiting till my stomach growls to eat my first meal
2. Only eating 1 meal and 1 tasting every day this week
3. Setting a timer for 10 minutes to make sure I'm eating slowly

---

1. Waiting to eat my first meal until noon.
2. Stop eating at a level 3.8
3. Cutting my portions in 1/2 and only eating 1/2 of what I normally eat

---

1. Only having 1 small sweet every day (like 8 M&Ms)
2. Doing a 24-hour fast
3. Waiting till my stomach growls and not eat before 1pm each day

---

1. Cutting creamer out of my coffee and doing a clean fast until I eat my first meal
2. Doing a 2-day fast
3. Setting a timer to make sure I take 20 minutes to eat my meal

---

1. Praying every time I'm tempted to eat when I'm not truly hungry and ask God to take the temptation away
2. Doing a 3-day fast
3. Working out 2 days a week

Write YOUR THREE Weekly Commitments Below:

1. _____

_____

2. _____

_____

3. _____

_____

Hunger Scale Accountability Chart

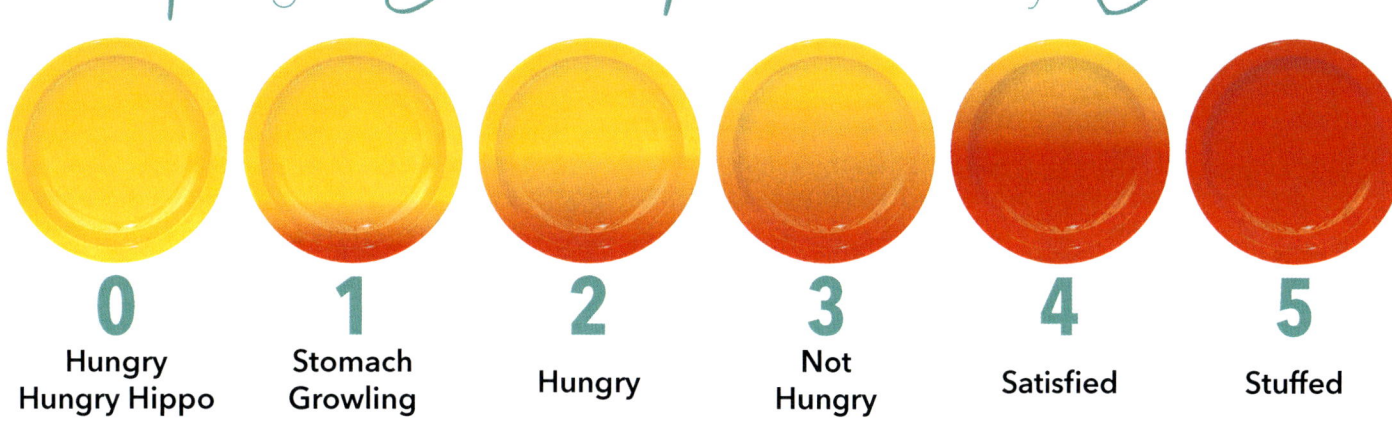

0	1	2	3	4	5
Hungry Hungry Hippo	Stomach Growling	Hungry	Not Hungry	Satisfied	Stuffed

	NOTE: Try and avoid the snack whenever possible.	Meal 1	Meal 2	Snack
Sample	Level When You Started Eating	1.3	2.0	
	Level When You Finished Eating	3.2	4.2	
DAY 1	Level When You Started Eating			
	Level When You Finished Eating			
DAY 2	Level When You Started Eating			
	Level When You Finished Eating			
DAY 3	Level When You Started Eating			
	Level When You Finished Eating			
DAY 4	Level When You Started Eating			
	Level When You Finished Eating			
DAY 5	Level When You Started Eating			
	Level When You Finished Eating			
DAY 6	Level When You Started Eating			
	Level When You Finished Eating			
DAY 7	Level When You Started Eating			
	Level When You Finished Eating			

End of Week Accountability Questions

1. Did you eat when you were at 0, 1, or 2 on the hunger scale and ask God for strength to wait till you reached one of those levels before eating? ○ Yes ○ No
2. Once you reached the point when your stomach was growling or was empty, did you eat foods that you love and that are 4 or 5 stars? ○ Yes ○ No
3. Did you stop before you were full at a level 4, and did you eat slowly in a non-stressful environment and savor your food? ○ Yes ○ No
4. Did you eat real foods without chemicals and limit sugar consumption? (Remember: None of the thin eaters counted carbs or removed sugar when they wanted to lose weight, but they did consciously limit sugar) ○ Yes ○ No
5. Did you eat when a stressful situation came up this week? ○ Yes ○ No
6. Did you eat for any other reason than true hunger this week? ○ Yes ○ No
7. Did you ever feel tired/sluggish after eating? ○ Yes ○ No

Friend Accountability Chart

Name	Email	Social Media Info	# of Times Contacted	Method Used

Weekly Accountability Chart

	Yes	No
Did you experience any temptation breakthroughs (like the cake story on page 43) this week or any time God provided a way out for you, so you didn't eat when you weren't hungry?		
Did you spend less time thinking about food?		
Are you starting to understand that you can eat what you want within your red, yellow, green light foods? (See page 80)		
Are you starting to eat ½ to ⅔ what you used to?		
Are you slowing down when you eat?		
Did you pick a fasting window and stick to it? (See page 30)		
Did you memorize any Bible verses to help you?		

Your Success Stories

It's important to celebrate your accomplishments! In *Fasting to Freedom*, I talk about enslaving sins. They cannot be fixed overnight. They take time to overcome. I cannot eat slowly; I've gotten better, but I'm not perfect. So I celebrate the other things I've learned to do well.

Rate how well you did (1-10) with these concepts over the past week:

Success	Rating
I tried an extended 24 hour fast	
I fasted longer than last week	
I put my fork down between each bite	
I cut my food portion in ½ or ⅓	
I did a quiet time every morning/night *Joshua 1:8* *Keep this Book of the Law always on your lips; meditate on it day and night, so that you may be careful to do everything written in it. Then you will be prosperous and successful.*	
I found an accountability partner to do an extended fast with me	
I ate the best foods on my plate first	
If I overate, I waited to do a 24-hour fast and got all the way to empty and hungry before eating again	
I ate more slowly than the day before	
I chose nutrient-dense foods	
I cut back on sugar	
I tried to eat more slowly	
I ate real foods without a lot of chemicals	

Success	Rating
I took smaller portions to begin with	
I asked the Holy Spirit to help me avoid eating when not hungry and to avoid false hunger	
I never ate beyond level 4 on the hunger scale	
I stopped eating at a 3.8 knowing that within 20 minutes I would be at a level 4	
I ate what I was craving instead of diet foods	
I only ate 1 or 2 meals a day and didn't fast	
I ate at a level 0, 1, or 2	
I prayed for discernment before I ate	
I didn't drink sweet beverages like sweet tea or sugary drinks or use gum/mints between mealtimes.	
I drank no calories drinks	

Weekly Prayer:

"God I want to get into a right relationship with food and only eat when I'm truly hungry and stop when I'm full. I never want to yo-yo diet again. Please let the Holy Spirit intervene whenever I'm about to overeat, and help so I **don't** overeat. Help me to slow down and savor my food and help me to fall in love with You, not food; let You be my fiancé and my go to, not the food." (See explanation on page 82)

Make your own prayer based on what you want to work on for the week:

_____

_____

_____

_____

Session 2:
The Shiny Ball Diet Syndrome

Weekly Ice Breaker

Peaks and Pits – Think about the past week. What were your Peaks and your Pits?

These can be food/eating-related but don't have to be. Your Peaks should be things that brought you joy, made you feel happy, made you smile, made you feel energized or excited – things you enjoyed and would enjoy doing again. Your Pits should be things that drained your energy, made you upset or angry, made you sad, made you frustrated, or gave you a headache – things you wish you didn't have to repeat again.

Now, write them in the spaces below:

Peaks	Pits

Weekly Game

Would You Rather. Put a piece of tape on the floor to separate the room in half. Rattle off a bunch of questions – e.g., would you rather travel to Italy or Australia? – everyone hops on either side of the line depending on their answer. It's an easy way to figure out what people have in common with one another.

Key Concepts

Proverbs 23:1-3
When you sit to dine with a ruler, note well what is before you,
and put a knife to your throat if you are given to gluttony.
Do not crave his delicacies, for that food is deceptive.

Fad diets will always be popular. The problem with them is that even though they address people's desire to lose weight quickly, they aren't sustainable for the long term. You must figure out something to do for life, and everyone who is mindlessly thin has figured out what works for them. Stop following all fad diets and eat real food! You may try to eat mindfully and with intention now, but be prepared to be tempted by fad diets. I call this the "Shiny Ball Diet Syndrome." This is my made up, fun phrase for describing when someone loses focus easily, as if a shiny ball rolls by and you go chase it no matter what else you are doing at the time. You have to pray to not be led astray by that shiny ball! Diets and restrictions are all part of the Shiny Ball Diet Syndrome designed to keep you in bondage. They limit what you can eat and force you to eat the same things over and over again until you just get sick of it. You want to eat what your body is craving. When you cut out so many foods, the more you can't have something, the more you think of it and become preoccupied with it. Why submit yourself to that bondage? Dieting–the practice of restricting what you can and can't eat–is slavery. It's creating a false god.

- Nutrisystem: low calorie, low fat, and nothing but processed foods
- Jenny Craig: low calorie, low fat and nothing but processed foods with tons of chemicals that you should not eat
- Atkins diet: low carb
- HCG diet: low cal, low carb, low fat
- Keto Diet: low carb, high fat
- Whole 30 diet
- Weight Watchers: counting points for everything that goes in your mouth
- Cabbage soup Diet
- South Beach Diet
- Slim Fast: "a shake for breakfast, another for lunch, and a sensible dinner"
- Suzanne Somers Diet
- Master Cleanse
- Elimination Diet
- Physician's Weight Loss Diet
- Grapefruit Diet

I've tried all of these, and they don't work because, though you may lose weight on them, you almost always gain it all back as soon as you come off the diet. They are not sustainable.

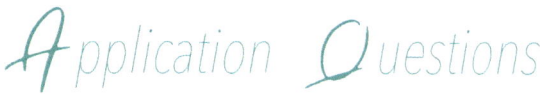

Application Questions

? Have you tried any other diets not on the list? Which?

_____

_____

As you scroll through social media you've probably seen many people boasting about some shiny new diet they're trying. Maybe you've even seen before and after pictures of their results. But remember, diets encourage you to eat certain foods like carrots or celery, even when you aren't physically hungry, which means you eventually return to weight gain when you fall off the diet wagon. *Freedom From Food* helps you recognize true physical hunger, helping you to prevent eating when you are not hungry.

SO I WILL REPEAT IT AGAIN: IF YOU ARE NOT PHYSICALLY HUNGRY, YOU DO NOT PUT A SINGLE BITE OF FOOD OR CALORIC DRINK IN YOUR MOUTH!!

Remember that diets cause you to lose, gain, lose, and gain back more weight, but they only highlight the losses, not the inevitable gains. With intermittent fasting, the weight comes off slower, but it *stays off*. That's the difference.

? Did you lose weight on a Shiny Ball Diet?

_____

? Did you gain the weight back?

_____

? What can you do to prevent yourself from falling for the Shiny Ball Diet Syndrome?

_____

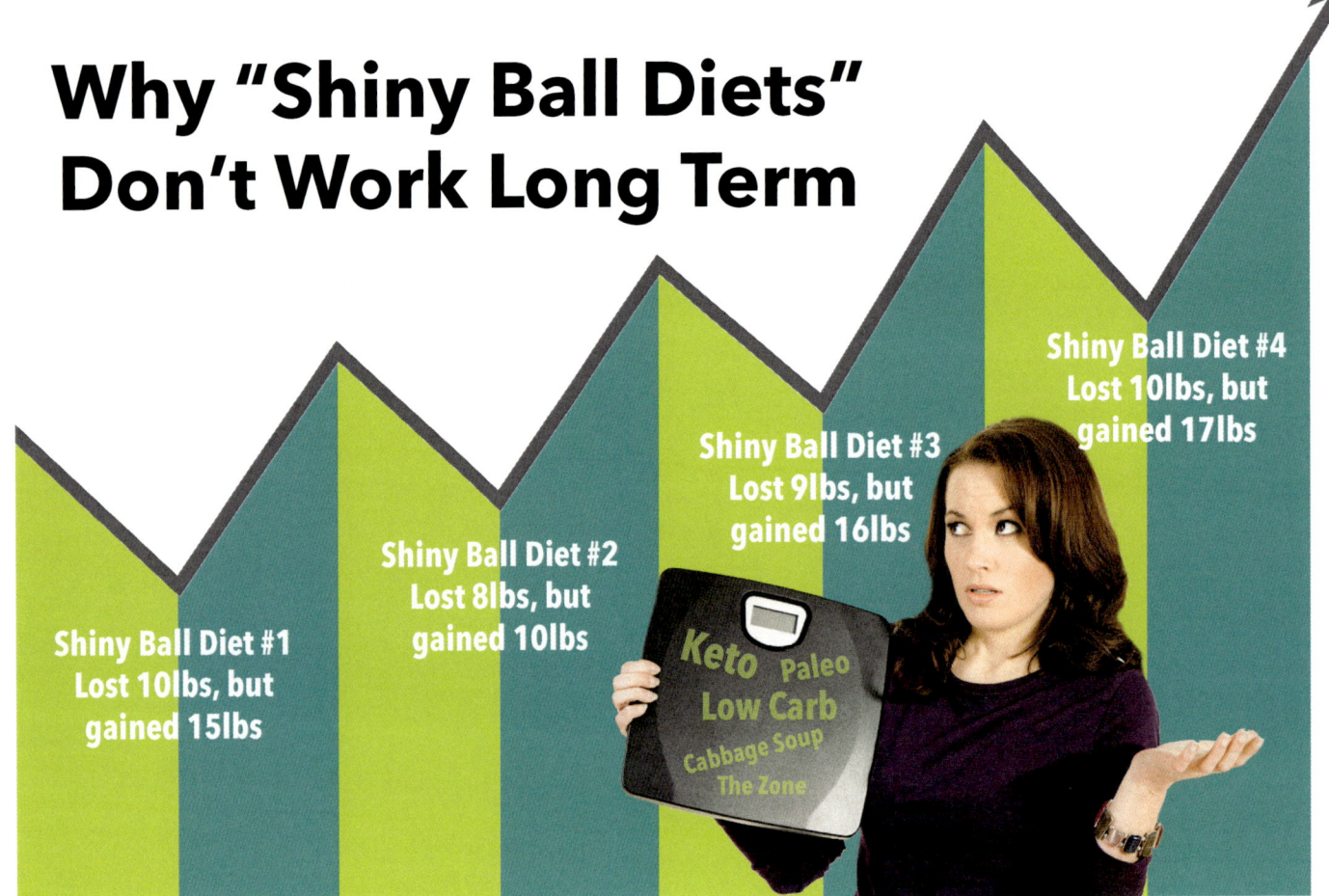

Why "Shiny Ball Diets" Don't Work Long Term

I just saw a friend of mine that I hadn't seen in about a year, and she had literally gained about 80 pounds in that one-year period. I asked, "Well, what are you doing these days?" She said, "Oh, I'm really happy. I'm doing the keto diet right now." This is exactly what I mean! You may initially lose weight on these Shiny Ball Diets, but eventually, you end up gaining even more back.

In today's world, almost everyone has a limited attention span. If a video or webpage doesn't load quickly enough, we give up and move on to the next thing. The key to success is for you to focus and keep your eye on the prize. Fasting isn't exciting. You won't get a new package in the mail every week filled with processed foods. This process is comparatively boring, but it works! Repeat after me: This program will result in slower weight loss than those Shiny Ball Diets, but this weight loss is *for life*.

Would you rather lose weight quickly on a Shiny Ball Diet and gain it all back, or go a little bit slower and be thin for life? I want you to ask yourself that question anytime the devil puts a Shiny Ball Diet in front of you. Ask yourself if you want to be all over again.

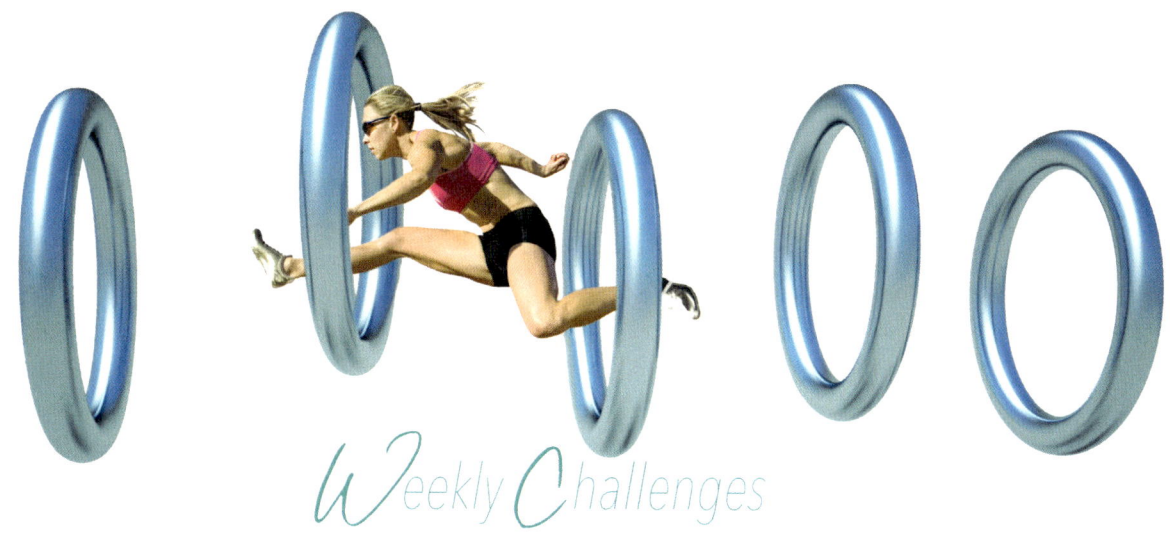

Weekly Challenges

A. Make *THREE NEW* Weekly Commitments:

❶ _____

_____

❷ _____

_____

❸ _____

_____

B. Meet With Your Accountability Partner at least once this week.

C. Weigh Yourself on Monday morning, and record your weight. Weigh yourself again on Sunday evening, and record your weight.

_____   _____
Monday Morning Weight   Sunday Night Weight

C. Use a Journal to record every time you eat when you're not truly hungry. See if you can find a pattern/ trigger.

D. Memory Verse:

Phillipians 3:14
I press on toward the goal to win the prize for which
God has called me heavenward in Christ Jesus.

Hunger Scale Accountability Chart

0	1	2	3	4	5
Hungry Hungry Hippo	Stomach Growling	Hungry	Not Hungry	Satisfied	Stuffed

	NOTE: Try and avoid the snack whenever possible.	Meal 1	Meal 2	Snack
Sample	Level When You Started Eating	1.3	2.0	
Sample	Level When You Finished Eating	3.2	4.2	
DAY 1	Level When You Started Eating			
DAY 1	Level When You Finished Eating			
DAY 2	Level When You Started Eating			
DAY 2	Level When You Finished Eating			
DAY 3	Level When You Started Eating			
DAY 3	Level When You Finished Eating			
DAY 4	Level When You Started Eating			
DAY 4	Level When You Finished Eating			
DAY 5	Level When You Started Eating			
DAY 5	Level When You Finished Eating			
DAY 6	Level When You Started Eating			
DAY 6	Level When You Finished Eating			
DAY 7	Level When You Started Eating			
DAY 7	Level When You Finished Eating			

End of Week Accountability Questions

1. Did you eat when you were at 0, 1, or 2 on the hunger scale and ask God for strength to wait till you reached one of those levels before eating? ○ Yes ○ No
2. Once you reached the point when your stomach was growling or was empty, did you eat foods that you love and that are 4 or 5 stars? ○ Yes ○ No
3. Did you stop before you were full at a level 4, and did you eat slowly in a non-stressful environment and savor your food? ○ Yes ○ No
4. Did you eat real foods without chemicals and limit sugar consumption? (Remember: None of the thin eaters counted carbs or removed sugar when they wanted to lose weight, but they did consciously limit sugar) ○ Yes ○ No
5. Did you eat when a stressful situation came up this week? ○ Yes ○ No
6. Did you eat for any other reason than true hunger this week? ○ Yes ○ No
7. Did you ever feel tired/sluggish after eating? ○ Yes ○ No

Friend Accountability Chart

Name	Email	Social Media Info	# of Times Contacted	Method Used

Weekly Accountability Chart

	Yes	No
Did you experience any temptation breakthroughs (like the cake story on page 43) this week or any time God provided a way out for you, so you didn't eat when you weren't hungry?		
Did you spend less time thinking about food?		
Are you starting to understand that you can eat what you want within your red, yellow, green light foods? (See page 80)		
Are you starting to eat ½ to ⅔ what you used to?		
Are you slowing down when you eat?		
Did you pick a fasting window and stick to it? (See page 30)		
Did you memorize any Bible verses to help you?		

Your Success Stories

It's important to celebrate your accomplishments! In *Fasting to Freedom*, I talk about enslaving sins. They cannot be fixed overnight. They take time to overcome. I cannot eat slowly; I've gotten better, but I'm not perfect. So I celebrate the other things I've learned to do well.

Rate how well you did (1-10) with these concepts over the past week:

Success	Rating
I tried an extended 24 hour fast	
I fasted longer than last week	
I put my fork down between each bite	
I cut my food portion in ½ or ⅓	
I did a quiet time every morning/night *Joshua 1:8* *Keep this Book of the Law always on your lips; meditate on it day and night, so that you may be careful to do everything written in it. Then you will be prosperous and successful.*	
I found an accountability partner to do an extended fast with me	
I ate the best foods on my plate first	
If I overate, I waited to do a 24-hour fast and got all the way to empty and hungry before eating again	
I ate more slowly than the day before	
I chose nutrient-dense foods	
I cut back on sugar	
I tried to eat more slowly	
I ate real foods without a lot of chemicals	

Success	Rating
I took smaller portions to begin with	
I asked the Holy Spirit to help me avoid eating when not hungry and to avoid false hunger	
I never ate beyond level 4 on the hunger scale	
I stopped eating at a 3.8 knowing that within 20 minutes I would be at a level 4	
I ate what I was craving instead of diet foods	
I only ate 1 or 2 meals a day and didn't fast	
I ate at a level 0, 1, or 2	
I prayed for discernment before I ate	
I didn't drink sweet beverages like sweet tea or sugary drinks or use gum/mints between mealtimes.	
I drank no calories drinks	

Weekly Prayer:

"God I want to get into a right relationship with food and only eat when I'm truly hungry and stop when I'm full. I never want to yo-yo diet again. Please let the Holy Spirit intervene whenever I'm about to overeat, and help so I **don't** overeat. Help me to slow down and savor my food and help me to fall in love with You, not food; let You be my fiancé and my go to, not the food." (See explanation on page 82)

Make your own prayer based on what you want to work on for the week:

_____

_____

_____

Session 3: Fasting

Weekly Ice Breaker

Peaks and Pits — Think about the past week. What were your Peaks and your Pits?

These can be food/eating-related but don't have to be. Your Peaks should be things that brought you joy, made you feel happy, made you smile, made you feel energized or excited — things you enjoyed and would enjoy doing again. Your Pits should be things that drained your energy, made you upset or angry, made you sad, made you frustrated, or gave you a headache — things you wish you didn't have to repeat again.

Now, write them in the spaces below:

Peaks	Pits

Weekly Game

Who is it? Each person writes down something about themselves that no one knows and puts it in a box. When everyone's done, the leader reads what's been written and the group tries to guess who did what.

What Is Intermittent Fasting?

Intermittent fasting is a pattern of eating in which you restrict the number of hours when you eat rather than track every calorie that you consume. In my own research I interviewed over 1,000 thin people and most of them did not have a specific hour of the day that they ate (e.g. lunch at 12, dinner at 6), but, just ate naturally based on when they were actually hungry. Most of them eat one or two meals a day in a window of time we call an eating window. You open your eating window when you consume your very first meal, snack, or caloric drink of the day; you close your eating window after you consume your very last calorie. When you're fasting, you can only drink water, coffee, and unsweetened tea.

There is no magic number of hours that every person should use for their eating window. Eight hours works great for some and six hours is better for others. Some people choose to eat only one meal and a snack a day in a window of four hours or fewer. The length of your eating window should be what works best for you with consideration of the portion sizes you eat.

Application Questions

? Have you ever tried Intermittent Fasting?

_____

? If so, what were your results?

_____

The basis of this lifestyle is this: don't restrict *what* you eat, but *when* you eat. You can eat what you like when you are physically hungry, as long as you only eat in your eating window and follow the FIRES Principles. These Principles work together with intermittent fasting. If you think you can lose weight by eating non-stop for eight hours straight, then you're sadly mistaken! FIRES will teach you to never overeat and to eat only when you're truly hungry. If your eating window is 8 hours long, then that means you're fasting for 16 hours. If you're eating for 6 hours, then you're fasting for 18. This is also called the clock approach. When using the clock approach, I recommend starting off with an 8-hour window while following the FIRES

Principles. If you don't see yourself losing weight, start reducing your window. The other way you can view intermittent fasting besides watching the clock is what I call the meal approach. The meal approach involves skipping one or two meals a day. If you want to melt fat away faster, look to the example of my many friends who only eat just one meal a day. The meal approach is great because you end up picking the meals that you want to eat each day with more intention.

The reason the number of hours you fast and eat have such a dramatic effect on your weight loss is because of how your body fuels itself. Your body has two options for fuel: glucose (sugar), from the food you recently ate, or fat that's already stored in your body. Your body will always burn sugar first. If there's so much sugar present that your body never needs to burn fat, you won't lose weight because fat-burning is what results in weight loss.

Imagine you have cash in your pocket and cash in the bank. You're not going to drive all the way to the bank to withdraw money if you have some already in your pocket. You're going to use up everything in your pocket first before you ever touch what's in the bank. That's how your body works with sugar (pocket money) and fat (money in the bank). After 18-24 hours of fasting, your body has burned up all of the sugar and starts attacking the fat. That's what you want! This is called transitioning from a sugar-burning mode to a fat-burning mode.

Application Questions

? Which approach do you think will work better for you, the clock approach or the meal approach?

___

? If you picked the clock approach, how long of an eating window would you try?

___

? If you chose the meal approach, which meal/meals would you eat?

___

Let's dive deep into how you've been doing with the principles you've learned over the last couple weeks. Answer these questions with as much detail as possible:

? Did you cut your portions down in ½ to ⅔ ? Why or why not?

_____

? Give examples of when you felt you had to eat everything on your plate.

_____

? Did you eat the very least amount to get yourself satisfied this week?

_____

? Before you put a single drop of food in your mouth, did you notice or ask yourself what level you were on the hunger scale?

_____

? Was there any point when you could've eaten a little bit less food and still have been satisfied?

_____

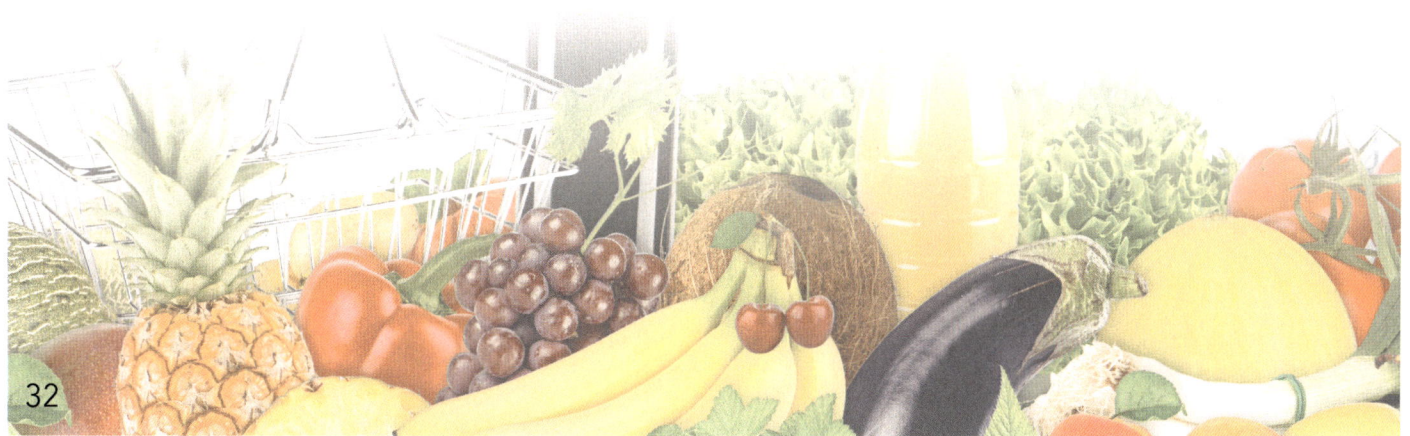

? Did you eat what you really really wanted every time? (Basically, did you become a Spice Girl and ask yourself, "Tell me what you want what you really, really want?")

? Even after I wrote my first book, *Waist Away: The Chantel Ray Way* (if you haven't read it, I strongly suggest you do because it really drives these principles home), I was still eating at certain times to a 4.1 or 4.2 on the Hunger Scale. Even on Thanksgiving, I never ate to a 5 or stuffed myself (though I don't really like turkey, cranberry sauce, pumpkin pie, or stuffing). In general, I wasn't overeating, and never ate past 4.4, but a lot of days I ate to 4.1, 4.2, 4.3, and I enjoyed it. I liked that feeling of just being a tiny bit past full, so I had to retrain my mind to get to a place where I enjoyed ending my meal at 3.8, 3.9, or 4.0. Was there ever a day you ate past level 4? If so, why?

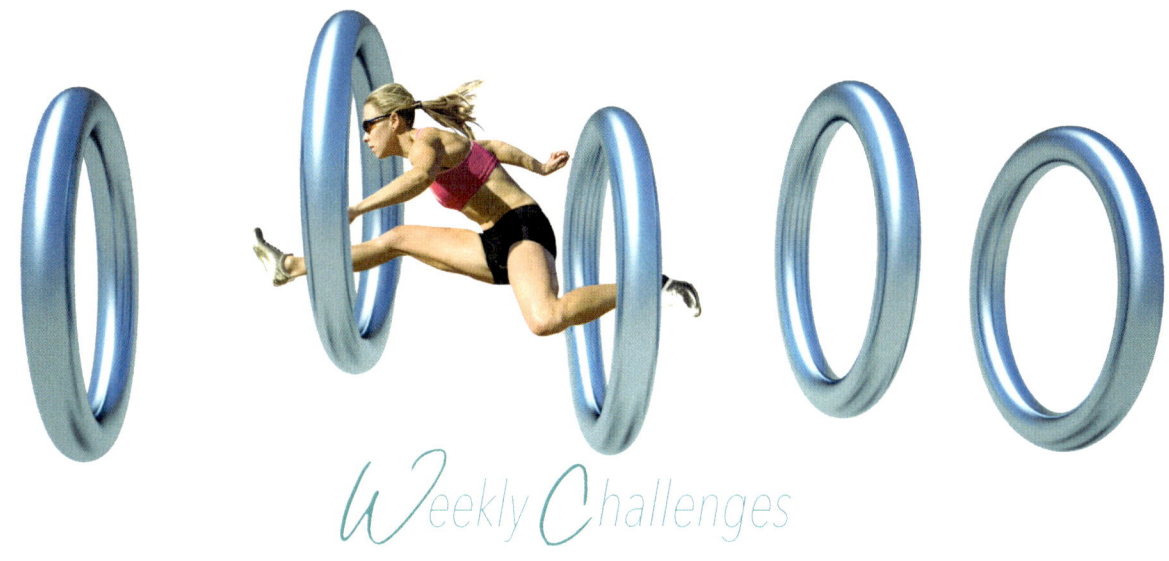

Weekly Challenges

A. Make *THREE NEW* Weekly Commitments:

① _____

_____

② _____

_____

③ _____

_____

B. Meet/Text With Your Accountability Partner at least once this week.

C. Weigh Yourself on Monday morning, and record your weight. Weigh yourself again on Sunday evening, and record your weight.

_____   _____
Monday Morning Weight   Sunday Night Weight

C. Use a Journal to record every time you eat when you're not truly hungry. See if you can find a pattern/ trigger.

D. Memory Verse:

Isaiah 58:6
Is not this the kind of fasting I have chosen: to loose the chains of injustice and untie the cords of the yoke, to set the oppressed free and break every yoke?

Hunger Scale Accountability Chart

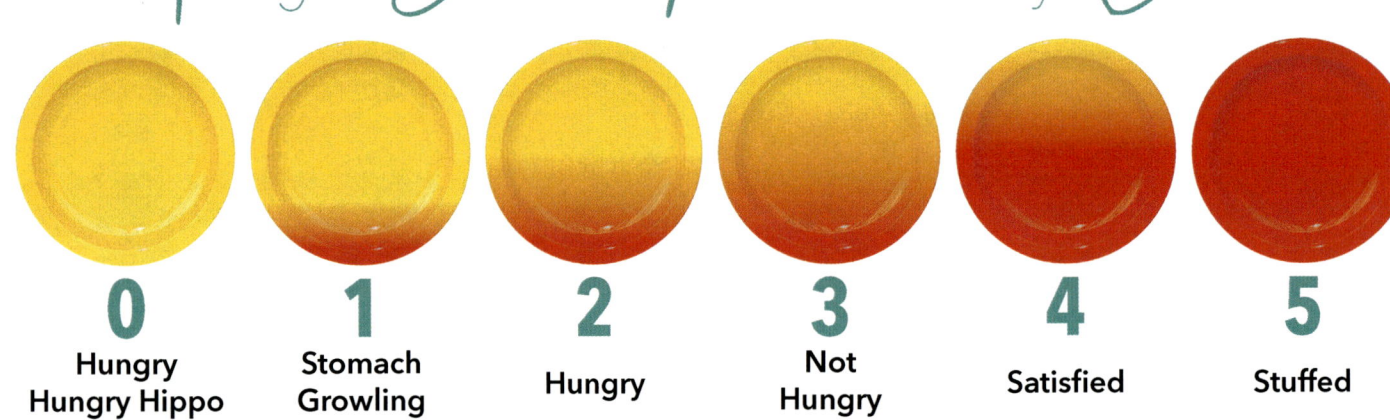

0	1	2	3	4	5
Hungry Hungry Hippo	Stomach Growling	Hungry	Not Hungry	Satisfied	Stuffed

	NOTE: Try and avoid the snack whenever possible.	Meal 1	Meal 2	Snack
Sample	Level When You Started Eating	1.3	2.0	
	Level When You Finished Eating	3.2	4.2	
DAY 1	Level When You Started Eating			
	Level When You Finished Eating			
DAY 2	Level When You Started Eating			
	Level When You Finished Eating			
DAY 3	Level When You Started Eating			
	Level When You Finished Eating			
DAY 4	Level When You Started Eating			
	Level When You Finished Eating			
DAY 5	Level When You Started Eating			
	Level When You Finished Eating			
DAY 6	Level When You Started Eating			
	Level When You Finished Eating			
DAY 7	Level When You Started Eating			
	Level When You Finished Eating			

End of Week Accountability Questions

1. Did you eat when you were at 0, 1, or 2 on the hunger scale and ask God for strength to wait till you reached one of those levels before eating? ○ Yes   ○ No
2. Once you reached the point when your stomach was growling or was empty, did you eat foods that you love and that are 4 or 5 stars? ○ Yes   ○ No
3. Did you stop before you were full at a level 4, and did you eat slowly in a non-stressful environment and savor your food? ○ Yes   ○ No
4. Did you eat real foods without chemicals and limit sugar consumption? (Remember: None of the thin eaters counted carbs or removed sugar when they wanted to lose weight, but they did consciously limit sugar) ○ Yes   ○ No
5. Did you eat when a stressful situation came up this week? ○ Yes   ○ No
6. Did you eat for any other reason than true hunger this week? ○ Yes   ○ No
7. Did you ever feel tired/sluggish after eating? ○ Yes   ○ No

Friend Accountability Chart

Name	Email	Social Media Info	# of Times Contacted	Method Used

Weekly Accountability Chart

	Yes	No
Did you experience any temptation breakthroughs (like the cake story on page 43) this week or any time God provided a way out for you, so you didn't eat when you weren't hungry?		
Did you spend less time thinking about food?		
Are you starting to understand that you can eat what you want within your red, yellow, green light foods? (See page 80)		
Are you starting to eat ½ to ⅔ what you used to?		
Are you slowing down when you eat?		
Did you pick a fasting window and stick to it? (See page 30)		
Did you memorize any Bible verses to help you?		

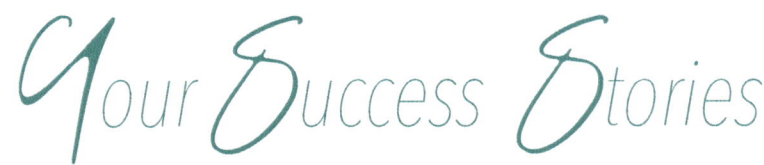

Your Success Stories

It's important to celebrate your accomplishments! In *Fasting to Freedom*, I talk about enslaving sins. They cannot be fixed overnight. They take time to overcome. I cannot eat slowly; I've gotten better, but I'm not perfect. So I celebrate the other things I've learned to do well.

Rate how well you did (1-10) with these concepts over the past week:

Success	Rating
I tried an extended 24 hour fast	
I fasted longer than last week	
I put my fork down between each bite	
I cut my food portion in ½ or ⅓	
I did a quiet time every morning/night *Joshua 1:8* *Keep this Book of the Law always on your lips; meditate on it day and night, so that you may be careful to do everything written in it. Then you will be prosperous and successful.*	
I found an accountability partner to do an extended fast with me	
I ate the best foods on my plate first	
If I overate, I waited to do a 24-hour fast and got all the way to empty and hungry before eating again	
I ate more slowly than the day before	
I chose nutrient-dense foods	
I cut back on sugar	
I tried to eat more slowly	
I ate real foods without a lot of chemicals	

Success	Rating
I took smaller portions to begin with	
I asked the Holy Spirit to help me avoid eating when not hungry and to avoid false hunger	
I never ate beyond level 4 on the hunger scale	
I stopped eating at a 3.8 knowing that within 20 minutes I would be at a level 4	
I ate what I was craving instead of diet foods	
I only ate 1 or 2 meals a day and didn't fast	
I ate at a level 0, 1, or 2	
I prayed for discernment before I ate	
I didn't drink sweet beverages like sweet tea or sugary drinks or use gum/mints between mealtimes.	
I drank no calories drinks	

Weekly Prayer:

"God I want to get into a right relationship with food and only eat when I'm truly hungry and stop when I'm full. I never want to yo-yo diet again. Please let the Holy Spirit intervene whenever I'm about to overeat, and help so I **don't** overeat. Help me to slow down and savor my food and help me to fall in love with You, not food; let You be my fiancé and my go to, not the food." (See explanation on page 82)

Make your own prayer based on what you want to work on for the week:

_____

_____

_____

_____

Session 4: Ways to Escape Temptation

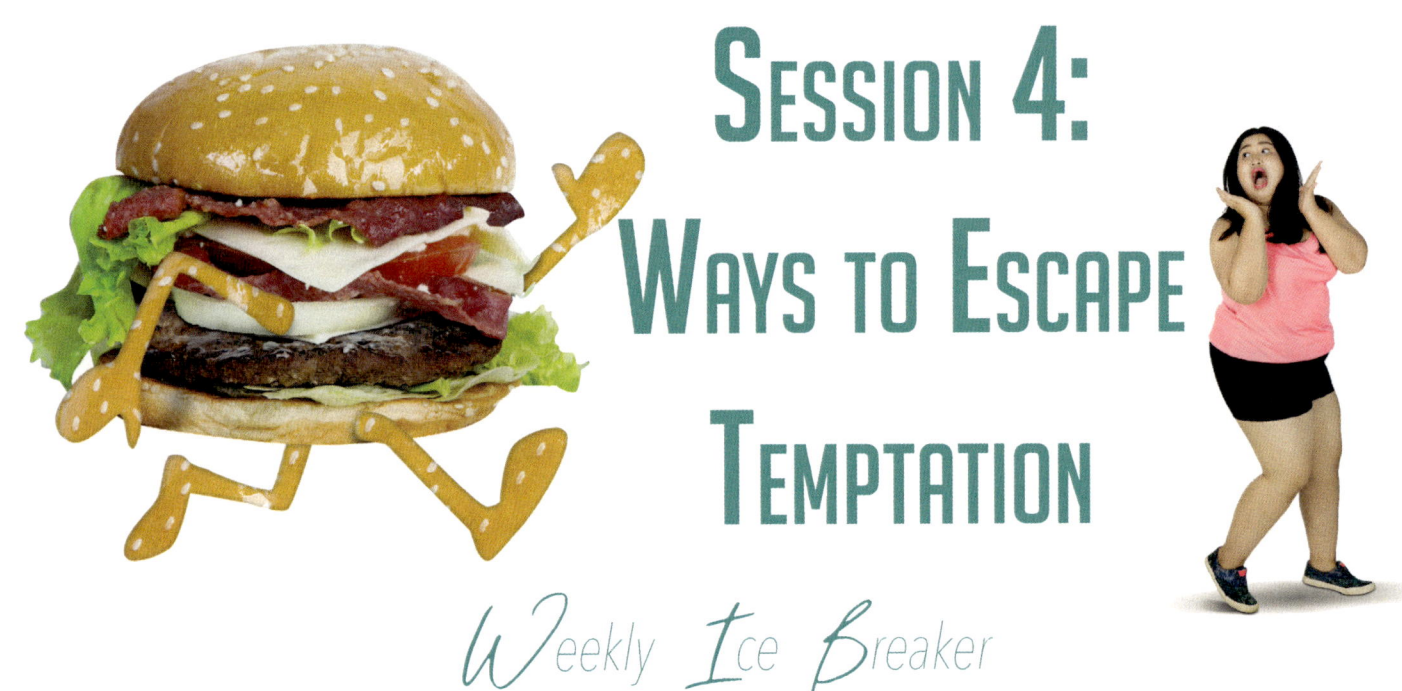

Weekly Ice Breaker

Peaks and Pits – Think about the past week. What were your Peaks and your Pits?

These can be food/eating-related but don't have to be. Your Peaks should be things that brought you joy, made you feel happy, made you smile, made you feel energized or excited – things you enjoyed and would enjoy doing again. Your Pits should be things that drained your energy, made you upset or angry, made you sad, made you frustrated, or gave you a headache – things you wish you didn't have to repeat again.

Now, write them in the spaces below:

Peaks	Pits

Weekly Game

Matchy Matchy. Before Bible Study begins, the leader writes a bunch of Bible verse addresses on sticky notes and then writes out the actual corresponding words of each verse on separate sticky notes. Then she mixes up the verse addresses and actual wording and sticks them all over the walls. The group must then go around the room and match the verse addresses to the correct corresponding verses written out. Whoever makes the most matches wins!

Bible Verse To Apply

Matthew 4:2-11

After fasting forty days and forty nights, he was hungry. The tempter came to him and said, "If you are the Son of God, tell these stones to become bread." Jesus answered, "It is written: 'Man shall not live on bread alone, but on every word that comes from the mouth of God.'"

Then the devil took him to the holy city and had him stand on the highest point of the temple. "If you are the Son of God," he said, "throw yourself down. For it is written: "'He will command his angels concerning you, and they will lift you up in their hands, so that you will not strike your foot against a stone.'"

Jesus answered him, "It is also written: 'Do not put the Lord your God to the test.'"

Again, the devil took him to a very high mountain and showed him all the kingdoms of the world and their splendor. "All this I will give you," he said, "if you will bow down and worship me."

Jesus said to him, "Away from me, Satan! For it is written: 'Worship the Lord your God, and serve him only.'" Then the devil left him, and angels came and attended him.

Application Question

The devil tempted Jesus with three things. What were they?

___

THE DEVIL HIMSELF QUOTED SCRIPTURE! The Devil will often twist Scripture and use it against us to tempt us.

SCENARIO: You're at party and not physically hungry, but your friend made a bunch of amazing food. The devil will quote things like 1 Peter 4:9 to you: "Offer hospitality to one another without grumbling," and you start to feel guilty that your friend made all this food, but no one is eating it. So how do you combat this??? **BY QUOTING SCRIPTURE!**

Times We Are Most Easily Tempted

Jesus countered Satan with "it is written" in the last two temptations just like He did in the first. The temptation may not leave immediately when you first quote a scripture verse, but that doesn't mean you stop. Sometimes you have to quote the Word multiple times. The weapons of the world are willpower, grit and determination. The weapons of the Christian believer have divine power! This is why we have to memorize Scripture. It's our divine weapon!!

Application Question

 Can you find any additional scriptures that deal with your recurring temptation? Which verse or verses?

_____

Before you make that wrong decision, attack the Devil with the Word.
"It is written …"
"It is written …"
"It is written …"
It may sound easy, but it's not easy when you're being tempted, and you feel weak. However, it's what Jesus did to fight Satan and it worked. You have two options: keep doing it your way (that doesn't work), or do it Jesus's way.

Luke 4:1-13

Jesus, full of the Holy Spirit, left the Jordan and was led by the Spirit into the wilderness, where for forty days he was tempted by the devil. He ate nothing during those days, and at the end of them he was hungry.

The devil said to him, "If you are the Son of God, tell this stone to become bread."

Jesus answered, "It is written: 'Man shall not live on bread alone.'"
The devil led him up to a high place and showed him in an instant all the kingdoms of the world. And he said to him, "I will give you all their authority and splendor; it has been given to me, and I can give it to anyone I want to. If you worship me, it will all be yours."

Jesus answered, "It is written: 'Worship the Lord your God and serve him only.'"
The devil led him to Jerusalem and had him stand on the highest point of the temple.

"If you are the Son of God," he said, "throw yourself down from here. For it is written:
"'He will command his angels concerning you to guard you carefully;
they will lift you up in their hands, so that you will not strike your foot against a stone.'"

Jesus answered, "It is said: 'Do not put the Lord your God to the test.'"
When the devil had finished all this tempting, he left him until an opportune time.

1. **When we are alone:** When we are lonely, it's easy to try to use anything to feel companionship, especially food.

2. **When we have just had a mountain top experience:** This happened right after Jesus was baptized and right after the Father in heaven said this is my beloved Son in whom I'm well pleased. We can often use food to feed a celebration, even if we are not physically hungry.

3. **When we are too hungry:** I know when I get too hungry, I can get tempted to overeat.

4. **When we are physically not feeling well or are sick:** This is my biggest one. Imagine when Jesus hadn't eaten for 40 days, I'm sure he didn't feel well! When I do a longer fast, I feel bad then start to feel better, but I can't imagine 40 days! I know I wouldn't feel well, would you?

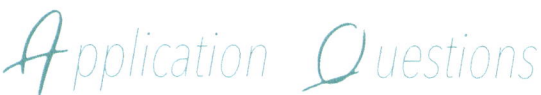

Which one of these four times is the most tempting for you?

Have you ever had a time where you were hit with temptation because you were too hungry?

Have you ever had a time where you were hit with temptation because you were lonely?

Have you ever had a time where you were hit with temptation after you had a mountain top experience?

The Cake Story

One of my friends, named Jo, makes a birthday cake that is absolutely to die for. It is perfectly moist, has whipped cream frosting, and layers of strawberries. For my daughter's 16th birthday, and we ordered a cake that was literally 3 feet by 2 feet! It was three times the size of what we needed. The kids ate none of it, so we were stuck with a ton leftover, and I found myself eating it for two days. One piece was on the counter next to the sink, and I was planning to eat it, even though I wasn't hungry, but I said that prayer: "God help me to not overeat." Then I accidentally ended up knocking the cake over into the sink full of dirty dishes. Even though it was an accident I started laughing and thanking God because I wasn't hungry and didn't want that cake after it had been in the sink with dirty dishes.

Application Question

? Can you name a time like this where you asked God to help you not overeat and the Holy Spirit intervened?

_____

God has a sense of humor and helps us with the little things in life. A lot of people think God is only concerned with big things, but that's not true! He wants to be a part of every little thing in your life including what you eat. This kind of relationship with God strengthens us as we learn to trust Him more and more. Involving him in what you eat is like inviting Him to your every meal! If you earnestly pray in the morning, "God protect me from myself, and make it so I don't eat these kinds of things," He will help you.

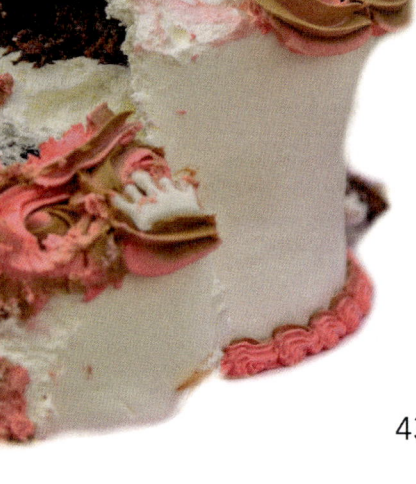

Application Questions

? What is your biggest food temptation?

___

? Are you more likely to resist or give into this temptation?

___

? How do you feel about your personal willpower? Is it strong or weak?

___

SHAM Acronym

SHAM is the acronym you can use to remember the times of highest temptation:

The devil is going to try to tempt you when you're:

S **Sick** *(Mentally and Physically)*

H **Hungry**

A **Alone**

M **Mountain Top Experience Finished**

1 Peter 5:8-9

Be alert and of sober mind. Your enemy the devil prowls around like a roaring lion looking for someone to devour. Resist him, standing firm in the faith, because you know that the family of believers throughout the world is undergoing the same kind of sufferings.

The devil is going to give you his shams. **Read Luke 4:3-4:**

The devil said to him, "If you are the Son of God, tell this stone to become bread."
Jesus answered, "It is written: 'Man shall not live on bread alone.'

What is the first temptation? Food! But Jesus replied, "Man shall not live on bread alone." Will you believe Satan's lie that over-fueling your body with food will give you the desire you want? It will never truly fill you up!

Read Luke 4:5-7:

The devil led him up to a high place and showed him in an instant all the kingdoms of the world. And he said to him, "I will give you all their authority and splendor; it has been given to me, and I can give it to anyone I want to. If you worship me, it will all be yours."

What is the second temptation? Power and excitement!

Read Luke 4:9-13:

The devil led him to Jerusalem and had him stand on the highest point of the temple.
"If you are the Son of God," he said, "throw yourself down from here. For it is written:
"'He will command his angels concerning you to guard you carefully;
they will lift you up in their hands, so that you will not strike your foot against a stone.'"
Jesus answered, "It is said: 'Do not put the Lord your God to the test.'"
When the devil had finished all this tempting, he left him until an opportune time.

❓ How will these Bible passages impact your life?

_____

_____

_____

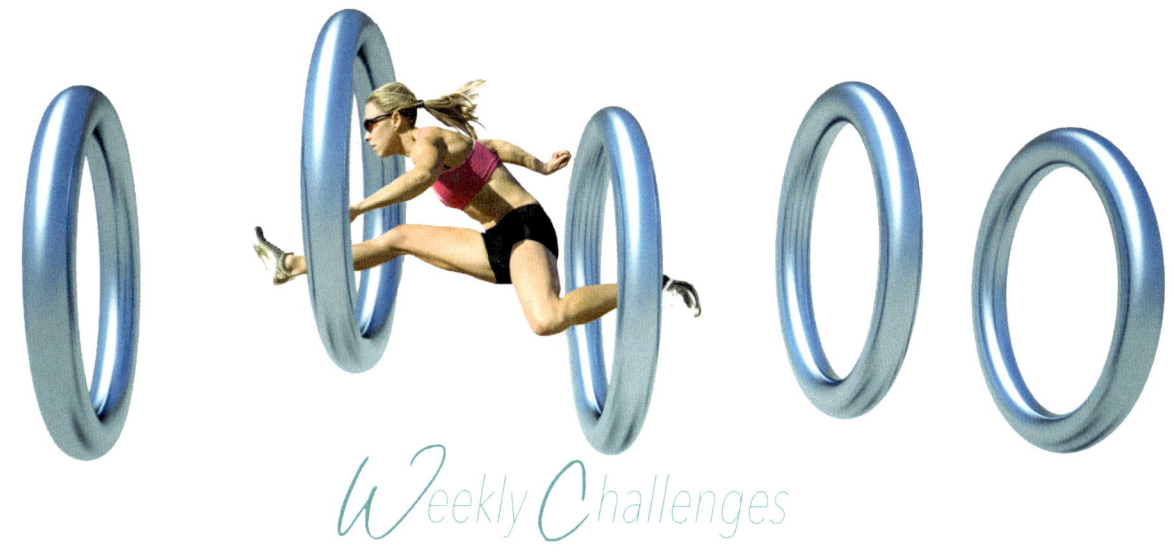

Weekly Challenges

A. Make *THREE NEW* Weekly Commitments:

❶ _____
_____

❷ _____
_____

❸ _____
_____

B. **Meet/Text With Your Accountability Partner** at least once this week.

C. **Weigh Yourself** on Monday morning, and record your weight. Weigh yourself again on Sunday evening, and record your weight.

_____   _____
Monday Morning Weight   Sunday Night Weight

C. **Use a Journal** to record every time you eat when you're not truly hungry. See if you can find a pattern/ trigger.

D. **Memory Verse:**

Matthew 4:4
Jesus answered, "It is written: 'Man shall not live on bread alone, but on every word that comes from the mouth of God.'"

Hunger Scale Accountability Chart

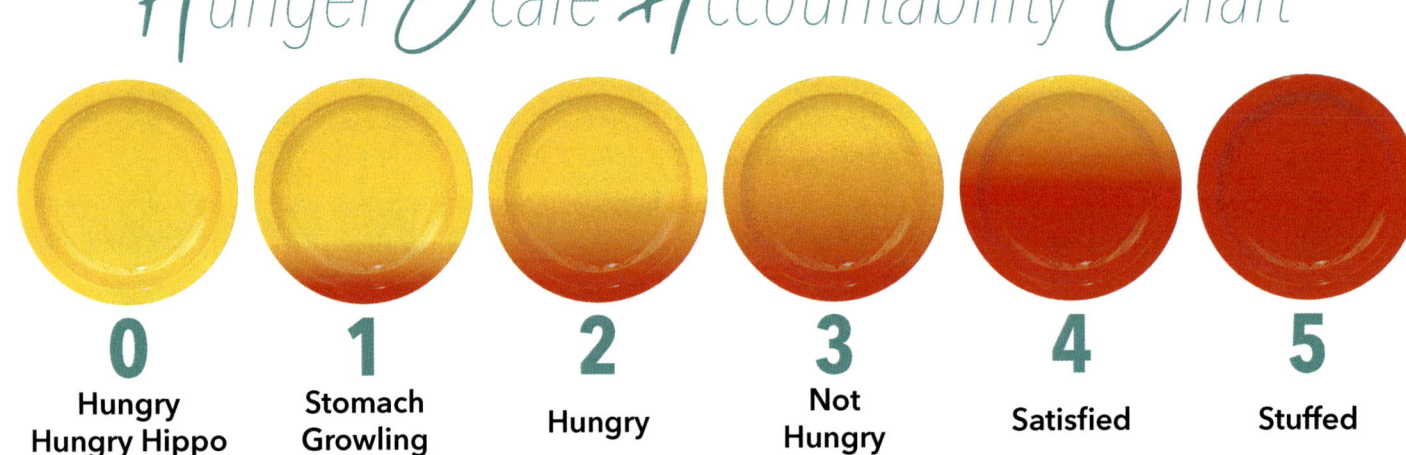

0	1	2	3	4	5
Hungry Hungry Hippo	Stomach Growling	Hungry	Not Hungry	Satisfied	Stuffed

	NOTE: Try and avoid the snack whenever possible.	Meal 1	Meal 2	Snack
Sample	Level When You Started Eating	1.3	2.0	
	Level When You Finished Eating	3.2	4.2	
DAY 1	Level When You Started Eating			
	Level When You Finished Eating			
DAY 2	Level When You Started Eating			
	Level When You Finished Eating			
DAY 3	Level When You Started Eating			
	Level When You Finished Eating			
DAY 4	Level When You Started Eating			
	Level When You Finished Eating			
DAY 5	Level When You Started Eating			
	Level When You Finished Eating			
DAY 6	Level When You Started Eating			
	Level When You Finished Eating			
DAY 7	Level When You Started Eating			
	Level When You Finished Eating			

End of Week Accountability Questions

1. Did you eat when you were at 0, 1, or 2 on the hunger scale and ask God for strength to wait till you reached one of those levels before eating? ○ Yes ○ No
2. Once you reached the point when your stomach was growling or was empty, did you eat foods that you love and that are 4 or 5 stars? ○ Yes ○ No
3. Did you stop before you were full at a level 4, and did you eat slowly in a non-stressful environment and savor your food? ○ Yes ○ No
4. Did you eat real foods without chemicals and limit sugar consumption? (Remember: None of the thin eaters counted carbs or removed sugar when they wanted to lose weight, but they did consciously limit sugar) ○ Yes ○ No
5. Did you eat when a stressful situation came up this week? ○ Yes ○ No
6. Did you eat for any other reason than true hunger this week? ○ Yes ○ No
7. Did you ever feel tired/sluggish after eating? ○ Yes ○ No

Friend Accountability Chart

Name	Email	Social Media Info	# of Times Contacted	Method Used

Weekly Accountability Chart

	Yes	No
Did you experience any temptation breakthroughs (like the cake story on page 43) this week or any time God provided a way out for you, so you didn't eat when you weren't hungry?		
Did you spend less time thinking about food?		
Are you starting to understand that you can eat what you want within your red, yellow, green light foods? (See page 80)		
Are you starting to eat ½ to ⅔ what you used to?		
Are you slowing down when you eat?		
Did you pick a fasting window and stick to it? (See page 30)		
Did you memorize any Bible verses to help you?		

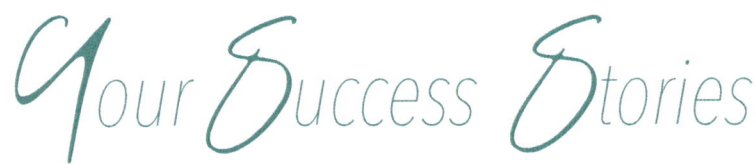

Your Success Stories

It's important to celebrate your accomplishments! In *Fasting to Freedom*, I talk about enslaving sins. They cannot be fixed overnight. They take time to overcome. I cannot eat slowly; I've gotten better, but I'm not perfect. So I celebrate the other things I've learned to do well.

Rate how well you did (1-10) with these concepts over the past week:

Success	Rating
I tried an extended 24 hour fast	
I fasted longer than last week	
I put my fork down between each bite	
I cut my food portion in ½ or ⅓	
I did a quiet time every morning/night *Joshua 1:8* *Keep this Book of the Law always on your lips; meditate on it day and night, so that you may be careful to do everything written in it. Then you will be prosperous and successful.*	
I found an accountability partner to do an extended fast with me	
I ate the best foods on my plate first	
If I overate, I waited to do a 24-hour fast and got all the way to empty and hungry before eating again	
I ate more slowly than the day before	
I chose nutrient-dense foods	
I cut back on sugar	
I tried to eat more slowly	
I ate real foods without a lot of chemicals	

Success	Rating
I took smaller portions to begin with	
I asked the Holy Spirit to help me avoid eating when not hungry and to avoid false hunger	
I never ate beyond level 4 on the hunger scale	
I stopped eating at a 3.8 knowing that within 20 minutes I would be at a level 4	
I ate what I was craving instead of diet foods	
I only ate 1 or 2 meals a day and didn't fast	
I ate at a level 0, 1, or 2	
I prayed for discernment before I ate	
I didn't drink sweet beverages like sweet tea or sugary drinks or use gum/mints between mealtimes.	
I drank no calories drinks	

Weekly Prayer:

"God I want to get into a right relationship with food and only eat when I'm truly hungry and stop when I'm full. I never want to yo-yo diet again. Please let the Holy Spirit intervene whenever I'm about to overeat, and help so I **don't** overeat. Help me to slow down and savor my food and help me to fall in love with You, not food; let You be my fiancé and my go to, not the food." (See explanation on page 82)

Make your own prayer based on what you want to work on for the week:

_____

_____

_____

_____

Session 5: 5 Ways to Q.U.I.E.T. the Devil

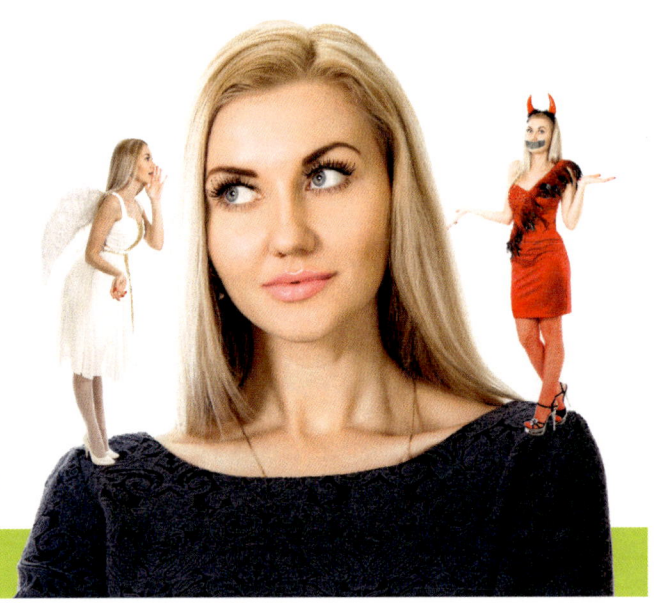

Weekly Ice Breaker

Peaks and Pits – Think about the past week. What were your Peaks and your Pits?

These can be food/eating-related but don't have to be. Your Peaks should be things that brought you joy, made you feel happy, made you smile, made you feel energized or excited – things you enjoyed and would enjoy doing again. Your Pits should be things that drained your energy, made you upset or angry, made you sad, made you frustrated, or gave you a headache – things you wish you didn't have to repeat again.

Now, write them in the spaces below:

Peaks	Pits

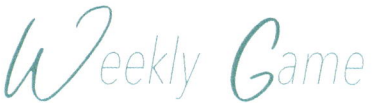

Weekly Game

Two Truths and a Lie: Ask all players to arrange themselves in a circle. Instruct each player to think of three statements about themselves related to food and/or eating. Two must be true statements, and one must be false. Each person then shares the three statements (in any order) with the group. The group votes on which one they feel is false, and at the end of each round, the person reveals which one was the lie.

Truth: _____

Truth: _____

Lie: _____

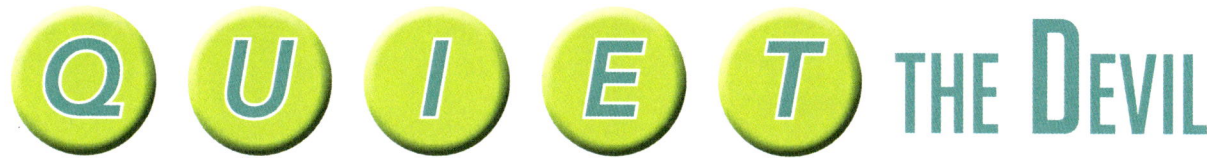

Quote Scripture:
Quote God's Word When You Want to Eat, but You're Not Hungry

You're going to experience great challenges as you desire to eat when you aren't truly hungry. You have to know how to fight temptations when they come. I want you to understand just how important God's Word is to the success of your fast.

Psalm 119:103
How sweet are your words to my taste, sweeter than honey to my mouth!

Substitute the Word of God in place of food. Suddenly, this verse takes on a new meaning because you're feasting on God's Word. His word is the best-tasting treat you could ever have in your mouth. You have to change your mindset because most people don't say, "Mmm, you know what I would love to have right now? A big dose of Psalms! I am really craving a big taste of Proverbs right now. I think I'm going to stop this car and read the book of Matthew right this second. I want it so bad that I can't even stand it!" Right? The Word of God is the answer when you need to find your way. It's the answer when you're weary and stressed out. There are blessings that come from seeking out the Word instead of other idols. There are so many things that God's Word does for you and it's truly the only thing you need.

Use the Holy Spirit:

Instead of relying on your self-discipline, you need to rely on God's discipline. Many of us were wrongly taught how to live the Christian life. I was taught about this "Christian Wheel" method when I first became a Christian. The idea was that if you wanted to be a good Christian there were certain things you had to do. You had to go to church every Sunday, pray, fellowship with other Christians, evangelize, and spend time in the Word of God. If you did those things, then you would have a fruitful Christian life. The part people miss is that you have to live your life through the power of the Holy Spirit. You have to do everything with the Lord's help. True Christian discipline sounds like this, "God, will you please help me get through this? I can't do this without you. I realize I am completely weak in this area. Without You, I can't turn from my old ways. I need Your help." Living your life with the help of the Holy Spirit is the only way to succeed. While all the things in that wheel are good, they're tools. They're not a substitute for the power of God. Pray and ask the Holy Spirit to grant you wisdom to make good choices and be balanced.

Identify Your True Feelings:

If you're not physically hungry but are drawn to eat for another reason, you need something besides food. For example, if you are lonely, you may need a hug; if you're feeling defeated at work, you may need reassurance; if you're feeling unloved by your husband, you may need love.

Four Ways to Stop Eating When You're Not Physically Hungry.

1. What are you really hungry for?

    Make a list (ex: affection, reassurance, friendship):

    _____

2. **Remind yourself of the consequences:** There are always consequences to sin; For example, if you eat an entire pan of brownies, you will feel physically awful and feel more uncomfortable, disappointed, and guilty than before you started, it's not worth it); think about the consequences of other sins.

    When I was 17 and had no money, my best friend and I loved expensive clothes, so we would go to Nordstrom and steal clothes. We did this for 8 months!! I was the best dressed 17 year old in Virginia. But one day we got caught, and after that point, I never stolen again. Now I'm fanatical about returning things, even little things like pens that I borrow.

    You must get to the point where you understand the consequences of overeating.

? Can you name a lesson you've learned from the consequences of a past sin??

_____

_____

_____

3. **Feed what you're truly longing for:**

   If you're lonely, call a friend, talk on the phone, or go to movie with someone. If you need friends, connect somewhere like a small group or Bible study; it takes work so take steps to make friends. If you're longing for a boyfriend, it takes effort. I get annoyed by my friends who constantly say they want a boyfriend, but when I ask if they're on any dating sites, they say no. Studies show that 93% of people are finding mates online. If 93% of all jobs were found on sites like Indeed and Monster, you'd be crazy not to use them to find a job! Even if dating sites aren't for you still must make the effort by joining a singles group at church or hanging out with single friends. Remember: If your fishing pole isn't in the water, you're not going to catch a fish. Don't complain but take no action. If you're feeling overwhelmed get in bath, go for walk, work out, meditate, do yoga, pray, listen to music, watch a favorite show. What's your favorite way to destress?

    How can you feed what you're actually hungry for?

   _____

4. **Identify your highest time or place of temptation.**

   For me, my highest time of temptation is when I don't feel well. I always think food will make me feel better, so I must spend more time with God instead and remind myself that if I'm not physically hungry, food won't help. You must figure out your highest temptation time. Is it when you're stressed?

   If I'm sick or stressed, I must remove snacks from the snack drawer behind my desk. Emotional eaters don't eat for hunger, they eat for every other reason, and can even overeat when they're happy. Awareness is key because emotional eating is mindless eating with food as your go-to. Some stress hormones make you crave sweet or salty foods (I'm one of those rare unicorns who doesn't discriminate and likes sweet and salty). A lot of non-Christian articles say that if you're stressed go for healthier options like rice cakes, carrots, or celery, but in my opinion if you're eating food when you're not physically hungry, you're sinning! (Reread the section on why overeating is a sin). Anytime an article says indulge in "healthy options", it's not from God. Does God ever encourage indulgence? The answer is no.

What is your go-to when you're stressed?

_____

 When is your highest time of temptation?

_____

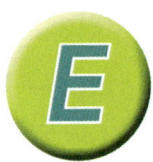 **Escape To A New Location:**

Step 1: Flee the scene of temptation immediately: My routine used to be that I would come home from school or work and have a snack. Now, I stay away from the kitchen when I get home, and I go do something else. If you're at a party with tempting food, don't stand next to the food table. Get yourself away from the scene of temptation.

Step 2: Remind yourself of your goal: Keep your eyes on the prize. Tell yourself that you're not eating until your stomach growls.

Step 3: Immediately pray and quote Bible verses: Jesus said that we live by the Word of God and not just bread (Matthew 4:4). Never depend on eating for joy and satisfaction.

Step 4: Find something else to do: Go for a walk, call a friend, do a puzzle, read a book. Do something that doesn't involve food. Start getting your mind off of your own desires. Ask yourself if you're actually hungry. Check to see if your stomach has even growled. Describe your symptoms of hunger and see if you're in the right spot on the Hunger Scale. True hunger is going to come approximately 1 to 2 times a day depending on how much you eat. You need to change your mindset and delight in being hungry.

List some other things you can do to avoid eating before you're truly hungry:

_____

_____

Talk To A Friend:

You don't have to stand up at work and yell out, "Hey everyone I'm struggling!" but you do need someone you can trust. You need someone who will love you, accept you, and pray for you without bringing you down. Don't lie to yourself and say you don't need help and that you don't really have a problem with food. The fact that you're afraid to admit your weakness in this area is what prevents you from going to the next level. Why do you think people don't want to share their problems with others? It's pride. Pride makes you insecure. Those secret sins in your life that you're embarrassed about aren't exclusive to you. I promise you, someone else is facing those exact same problems! In fact, God wants us to help each other with these problems.

Weekly Challenges

A. Make *THREE NEW* Weekly Commitments:

1. _____

2. _____

3. _____

B. Meet/Text With Your Accountability Partner at least once this week.

C. Weigh Yourself on Monday morning, and record your weight. Weigh yourself again on Sunday evening, and record your weight.

_____   _____
Monday Morning Weight   Sunday Night Weight

C. Use a Journal to record every time you eat when you're not truly hungry. See if you can find a pattern/ trigger.

D. Memory Verse:

1 Corinthians 10:13

No test or temptation that comes your way is beyond the course of what others have had to face. All you need to remember is that God will never let you down; he'll never let you be pushed past your limit; he'll always be there to help you come through it.

Hunger Scale Accountability Chart

0 — Hungry Hungry Hippo
1 — Stomach Growling
2 — Hungry
3 — Not Hungry
4 — Satisfied
5 — Stuffed

	NOTE: Try and avoid the snack whenever possible.	Meal 1	Meal 2	Snack
Sample	Level When You Started Eating	1.3	2.0	
	Level When You Finished Eating	3.2	4.2	
DAY 1	Level When You Started Eating			
	Level When You Finished Eating			
DAY 2	Level When You Started Eating			
	Level When You Finished Eating			
DAY 3	Level When You Started Eating			
	Level When You Finished Eating			
DAY 4	Level When You Started Eating			
	Level When You Finished Eating			
DAY 5	Level When You Started Eating			
	Level When You Finished Eating			
DAY 6	Level When You Started Eating			
	Level When You Finished Eating			
DAY 7	Level When You Started Eating			
	Level When You Finished Eating			

End of Week Accountability Questions

1. Did you eat when you were at 0, 1, or 2 on the hunger scale and ask God for strength to wait till you reached one of those levels before eating? ○ Yes ○ No
2. Once you reached the point when your stomach was growling or was empty, did you eat foods that you love and that are 4 or 5 stars? ○ Yes ○ No
3. Did you stop before you were full at a level 4, and did you eat slowly in a non-stressful environment and savor your food? ○ Yes ○ No
4. Did you eat real foods without chemicals and limit sugar consumption? (Remember: None of the thin eaters counted carbs or removed sugar when they wanted to lose weight, but they did consciously limit sugar) ○ Yes ○ No
5. Did you eat when a stressful situation came up this week? ○ Yes ○ No
6. Did you eat for any other reason than true hunger this week? ○ Yes ○ No
7. Did you ever feel tired/sluggish after eating? ○ Yes ○ No

Friend Accountability Chart

Name	Email	Social Media Info	# of Times Contacted	Method Used

Weekly Accountability Chart

	Yes	No
Did you experience any temptation breakthroughs (like the cake story on page 43) this week or any time God provided a way out for you, so you didn't eat when you weren't hungry?		
Did you spend less time thinking about food?		
Are you starting to understand that you can eat what you want within your red, yellow, green light foods? (See page 80)		
Are you starting to eat ½ to ⅔ what you used to?		
Are you slowing down when you eat?		
Did you pick a fasting window and stick to it? (See page 30)		
Did you memorize any Bible verses to help you?		

Your Success Stories

It's important to celebrate your accomplishments! In *Fasting to Freedom*, I talk about enslaving sins. They cannot be fixed overnight. They take time to overcome. I cannot eat slowly; I've gotten better, but I'm not perfect. So I celebrate the other things I've learned to do well.

Rate how well you did (1-10) with these concepts over the past week:

Success	Rating
I tried an extended 24 hour fast	
I fasted longer than last week	
I put my fork down between each bite	
I cut my food portion in ½ or ⅓	
I did a quiet time every morning/night *Joshua 1:8* *Keep this Book of the Law always on your lips; meditate on it day and night, so that you may be careful to do everything written in it. Then you will be prosperous and successful.*	
I found an accountability partner to do an extended fast with me	
I ate the best foods on my plate first	
If I overate, I waited to do a 24-hour fast and got all the way to empty and hungry before eating again	
I ate more slowly than the day before	
I chose nutrient-dense foods	
I cut back on sugar	
I tried to eat more slowly	
I ate real foods without a lot of chemicals	

Success	Rating
I took smaller portions to begin with	
I asked the Holy Spirit to help me avoid eating when not hungry and to avoid false hunger	
I never ate beyond level 4 on the hunger scale	
I stopped eating at a 3.8 knowing that within 20 minutes I would be at a level 4	
I ate what I was craving instead of diet foods	
I only ate 1 or 2 meals a day and didn't fast	
I ate at a level 0, 1, or 2	
I prayed for discernment before I ate	
I didn't drink sweet beverages like sweet tea or sugary drinks or use gum/mints between mealtimes.	
I drank no calories drinks	

Weekly Prayer:

"God I want to get into a right relationship with food and only eat when I'm truly hungry and stop when I'm full. I never want to yo-yo diet again. Please let the Holy Spirit intervene whenever I'm about to overeat, and help so I **don't** overeat. Help me to slow down and savor my food and help me to fall in love with You, not food; let You be my fiancé and my go to, not the food." (See explanation on page 82)

Make your own prayer based on what you want to work on for the week:

_____

_____

_____

Session 6: The All or Nothing Mentality

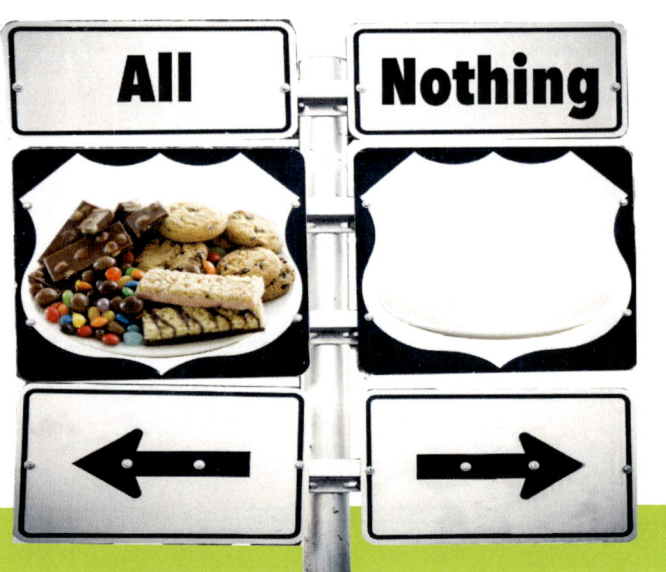

Weekly Ice Breaker

Peaks and Pits – Think about the past week. What were your Peaks and your Pits?

These can be food/eating-related but don't have to be. Your Peaks should be things that brought you joy, made you feel happy, made you smile, made you feel energized or excited – things you enjoyed and would enjoy doing again. Your Pits should be things that drained your energy, made you upset or angry, made you sad, made you frustrated, or gave you a headache – things you wish you didn't have to repeat again.

Now, write them in the spaces below:

Peaks	Pits

Weekly Game

Personal Scavenger Hunt: Break the group into two teams. Have everyone take out their phones. The leader tells everyone to look in their saved pictures for each item on a list, one at a time:

- A picture of a baby
- A picture of spaghetti
- A picture of someone else's children
- A picture of the beach
- A picture of a Christmas tree

Whichever team finds the picture first gets a point. Whichever team has the most points at the end, wins!

Titus 2:11-12
For the grace of God has appeared that offers salvation to all people. It teaches us to say "No" to ungodliness and worldly passions, and to live self-controlled, upright and godly lives in this present age.

Key Concepts

One of things I hear people say a lot is, "It's all or nothing for me when it comes to food. I can't even have one chip because if I do, I'll eat them all. Or, "If I eat one M&M, I'll eat the whole bag." The problem is that by depriving yourself of these things, eventually you will give in and end up overeating. You must allow yourself to have some. If you keep this all or nothing mentality, eventually you will go to a party, lose your mind, and overeat. You can retrain yourself to eat just ½ a candy bar or 3 chips, or just have a little and save the rest for later. That's what we are learning in this Bible Study. Instead of relying on your self-discipline, you need to rely on God's discipline.

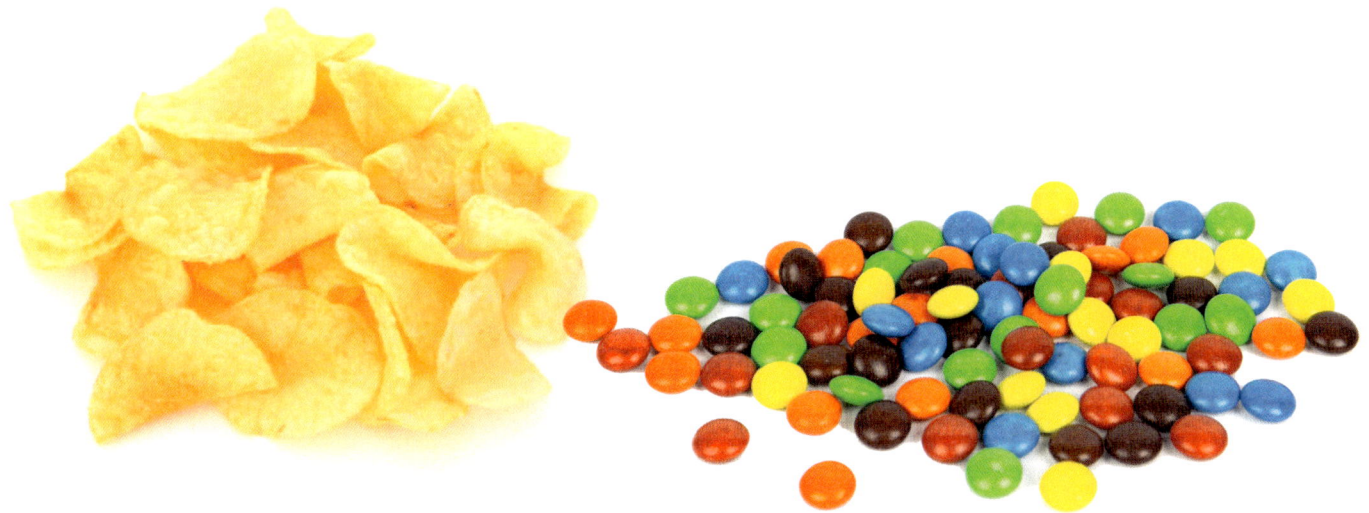

Application Questions

? What's your favorite thing to eat?

_____

? What do you deprive yourself of because you can't control yourself?

_____

When You're Skating on the Edge of Temptation, Try to Get Rid of the Pull of the Forbidden:

One girl in Bible study said, "When I eat potato chips, I always eat too many, so I avoid them like the plague!" Have you ever had thoughts like that? I'm against depriving yourself of any foods because it eventually makes you overeat those foods. She even admitted that she overeats them because she feels deprived. If I have a problem food, like chips, I actually eat them more often but in smaller quantities. For example, I put seven chips in a baggy and eat them at lunch and dinner to retrain my body. Seven chips won't make me fat, and this removes the pull of forbidden food.

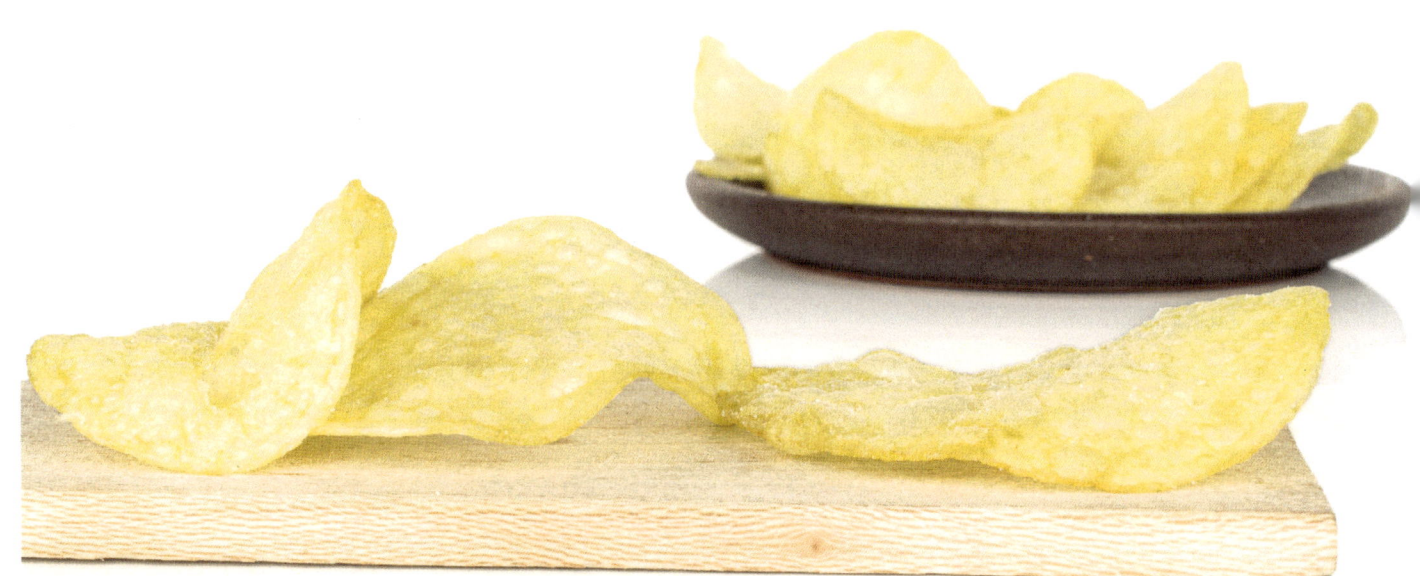

Tips To Not Overeat

One of things that I have heard a lot of the thin eaters say is that they like to drink wine. A lot of them stop at a 1 or 2 on the Hunger Scale after dinner, but they save room for wine and dessert. Also, a lot of times, they might have wine, but not dessert. Many say they stop eating at 3.6 or 3.5 on the Hunger Scale because they know they're going to drink wine or have some kind of chocolate. One of my friends, Allison always carries Hershey's kisses in her purse. Hershey's kisses are only about 20 calories each, so when she has 1 or 2, she feels satisfied because she had chocolate. Another friend, Debb always carries mini peppermint patties with her. Mini peppermint patties are only about 50 calories each, and one satisfies her and cuts her cravings.

Another tip to not overeating is making sure you eat what you want *first*. One time I went to Pollard's Chicken and saw a woman eat chocolate cake first and then eat the chicken. She was very thin. She said she didn't want to overeat but knew she wanted cake, so she had four bites of that first. Another thin eater got an ice cream sundae and ate it first because she knew she couldn't take that home without it melting, then she ate ½ of her food and took the rest home to eat the next day.

Application Questions

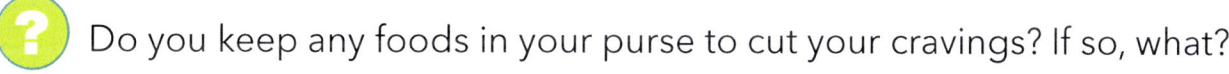

Do you keep any foods in your purse to cut your cravings? If so, what?

_____

Do you ever eat dessert first?

_____

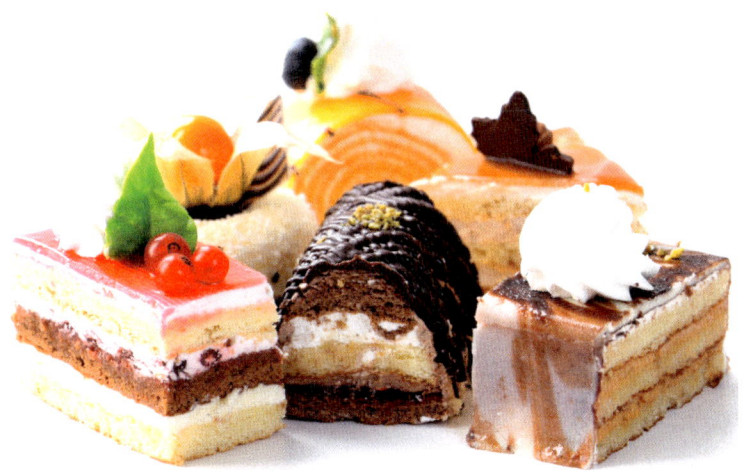

Physically Full vs Mentally Satiated

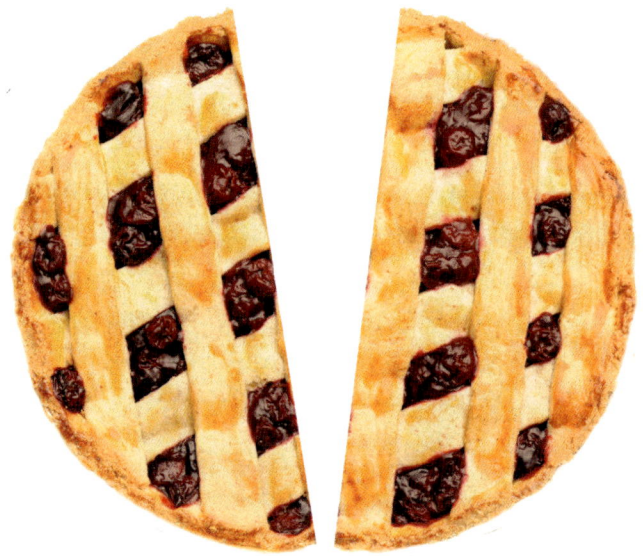

Picture a pie:
½ the pie is Physical Fullness, and the other ½ is Mental Satiety.

Burrito Story

A girl in Bible Study told me she'd wanted a bean burrito but looked at the Nutrition Facts and saw that it had 97 grams of carbs, so she decided not to have it and made a huge salad instead. After she ate the salad though, she still wanted the burrito, so she ate it anyway. I hear this same story over and over again. Why? Because of the pie principle. Are you physically full? Yes, but if you're not mentally satiated, you will continue to eat and focus on what you're actually craving. She should have had ½ the burrito to begin with. If you want the burrito, eat the burrito!

Application Questions

? Name a time you didn't eat what you were craving because you thought it wasn't healthy and then ended up overeating something else or eating something else plus the thing you were craving in the first place:

_____

_____

_____

You need to start eating what you want and not what you think you should eat. One time I went to lunch with my friend, Allison. I don't eat pizza very often, but that day I was craving pizza, so we went to Uno's Pizzeria and Grill. I ordered a small personal-sized pan pizza with onions pepperoni, and veggies. Allison said, "Mmm that pizza sounds tasty, but I'm going to be good and just get the grilled chicken Caesar salad." Well her salad came out, and the plate was literally a foot long. It was huge! It had tons of Caesar dressing, croutons, grilled chicken, and Parmesan cheese. If you look up the calories in a Caesar salad that size, it's at least 1000 to 1200, but in her mind, Allison thought she was "being good" by ordering the salad, even though she thought the pizza sounded good. Meanwhile, I ate half of my personal-sized pizza and was satisfied and planned to just save the other half. Well, after Allison finished her salad, she saw my leftover pizza and said, "I tried to be good with the salad, but I really want pizza. Can I have the rest of yours?" So, she ended up eating her entire salad plus half of my pizza. This is exactly what a lot of people with a weight problem do; they order what they think is better for them or healthier, but it's not what they really want, so they end up eating that *plus* what they really want. Allison would have been better off just ordering the pizza in the first place because it was what she really wanted. Cheese pizza from the average restaurant is 950 calories, while a Caesar salad can be as much as 1280 calories. Crazy, right? You can get so caught up on trying to eat healthfully and think you're doing well, when really, you're missing out on eating what you really want, and there's no reason for it. So I'll say it again:

Eat What You Really Want!

Get Out of the Clean Plate Club

Did you have a "food pusher" in your family? Someone who was always encouraging you to eat more, or finish this or try that? Was it your mom, dad, grandmother? Did you have someone who told you that you must finish your plate because children were starving in other countries, so you shouldn't waste food? Repeat after me: You are allowed to waste food!! You can either waste it in the trash or waste it on your hips.

Application Questions

? Who were the food pushers in your family?

_____

? Do they still pressure you to eat when you aren't hungry?

_____

Just Enough

One of the things all the thin eaters told me was that they like to stop eating as soon as they had "just enough." Just enough is right before you're full. The slower you eat the easier it is to gauge when you get "just enough." I do really well with almost all the thin eating concepts, but I have the hardest times with eating slowly. This is hard for me because I do everything quickly. One thing that helps me is to find distractions to help me slow down like doing work while I eat or stopping and talking to someone else while I eat.

All the thin eaters said:
(make these a mantra)

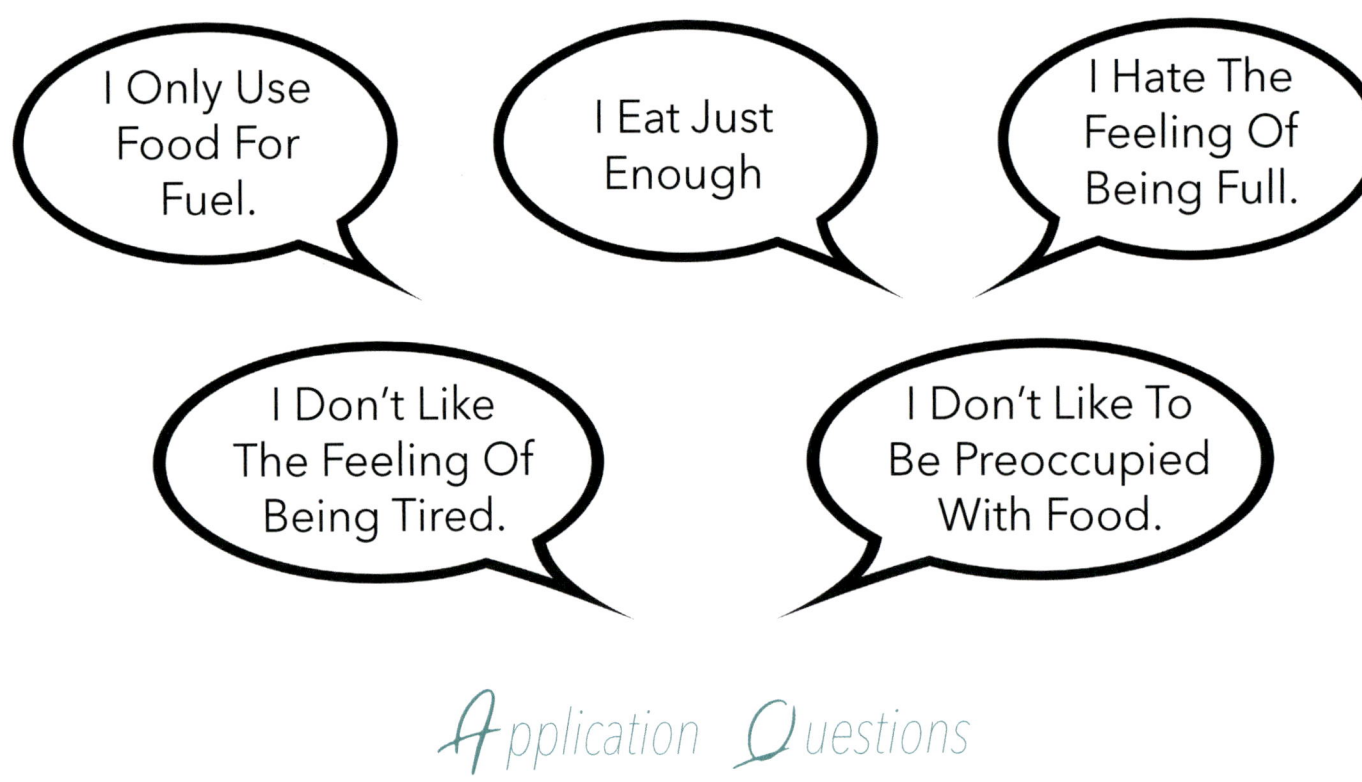

Application Questions

? Name some things you can do to help you recognize when you've eaten just enough:

_____

_____

One of my favorite restaurants is called Café Rio but I don't get it often because it's about 45 minutes away, so I recently had a friend deliver me a salad from there.

Here are a couple of tidbits from eating that salad that show you how to eat just enough:

> a) I picked out all my favorite parts of the salad first. I love cilantro, so I ate all of that and the lettuce but left most of the chicken and rice.
>
> b) I planned to go for a walk after I ate and didn't want to eat too much. A good way to gauge whether you ate too much is whether you can go for a walk right after you eat. You should be able to.

When most people who are trying to lose weight start to eat, they go straight for what they think should eat, like the vegetables, but they should go for what they love the most first! This is so important because if you start with the vegetables and fill up on them, you will be physically full, but not satiated. And, even though you are already full, you will still probably end up eating the things you like the best to feel mentally satiated.

I cannot stress this enough: Eat what really want and make sure it matches my 5-Star Enjoyment Scale!

> ★: Not Very Good
> ★ ★: Ehh
> ★ ★ ★: Pretty Good
> ★ ★ ★ ★: Party in My Mouth
> ★ ★ ★ ★ ★: Best Thing I've Ever Had

On a scale of 1-5, you want to only eat foods that are a 4-5 level of enjoyment. You shouldn't even waste calories on anything beneath that. If the steak and potatoes are your 5s, eat them first. Once you're full, you don't have to eat anything more. You're done!

Application Question

? Name some of your 5-Star foods.

You just want to remember to rate your foods and only eat what you really want. If someone brought in blueberry muffins and someone else brought in Krispy Kreme donuts, I would want the muffin. However, I would only eat the muffin top because that's my highest rated thing. Just eat the best things!

Thin eaters only eat what they really, really love. I interviewed tons of thin eaters and they told me that they actually taste and rate each food on their plates. The average eater tastes something she doesn't like and eats it anyway because she feels she has to "clean her plate."

1. Imagine a plate of steak, mashed potatoes, broccoli, and a salad. The average eater eats the foods she likes least first and saves the best for last. The thin eater eats whatever she likes the best first because she knows that she's going to stop eating once she gets full. If she likes the steak and mashed potatoes, she's going to eat that instead of feeling forced to eat the broccoli and salad she doesn't want. She eats what she craves.

2. Usually, a salad is served before the main course of any meal and we eat it not because we enjoy it, but because it's there. When the main course comes out—and, be honest, that's the food you showed up for—you eat more of that to satisfy your craving and end up eating past full. Afterward, you blame it on the meat and carbs in the main course when it's actually the salad that's the problem. You could have refused to eat that entirely and waited on what you actually wanted and eaten less overall.

3. Start rating not just the foods on your plate, but even the parts of each food. I like edges of brownies instead of the middle. So, I should just eat the edges. I don't have to eat the whole thing, just the best part. This is why thin eaters always leave some food on their plates. They are not part of the "clean your plate" club.

4. To make sure that you're only eating what you really want, use the enjoyment scale.

Application Question

? Using the Enjoyment Scale, rate the following foods:

Broccoli: _____

Donuts: _____

Chocolate Cake: _____

Salad: _____

Steak: _____

Potato Chips: _____

four Phases of freedom from food

1. **Complete food freedom:** no more fad diets or counting calories

2. **Discernment not Deprivation:** discern which foods make you feel your best

3. **Chose red-light, yellow-light, green-light foods:** decide which foods you can eat anytime, which you should limit, and which you should avoid to help you feel your best

4. **Maintenance:** maintain your healthy lifestyle and sustain your weight loss

Application Question

? Watch the video at chantelrayway.com/biblestudy called, "How do you determine hunger?" What did it teach you about understanding true hunger?

___

___

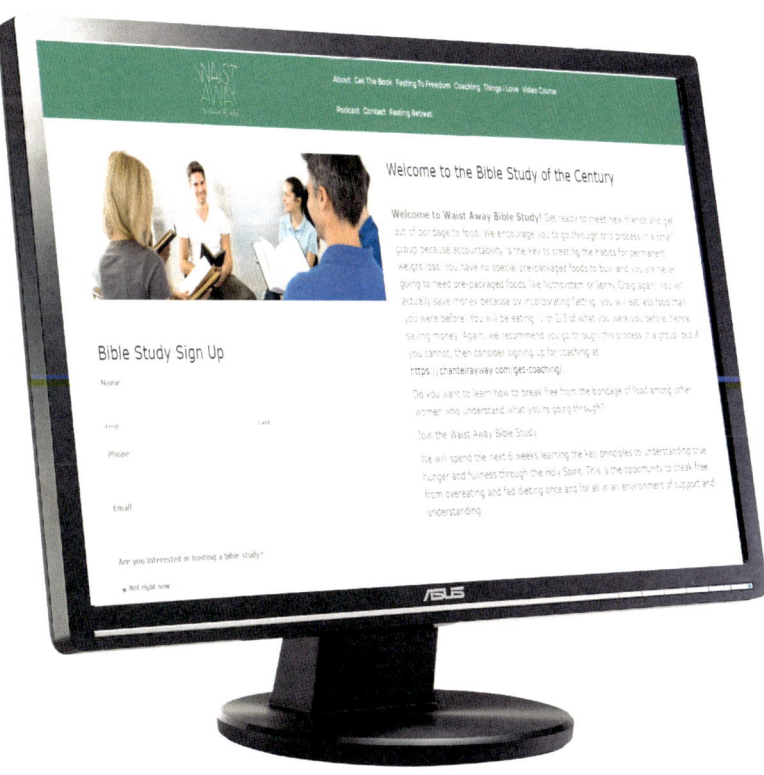

Restoration Through Jesus

Luke 8:26-39

They sailed to the region of the Gerasenes, which is across the lake from Galilee. When Jesus stepped ashore, he was met by a demon-possessed man from the town. For a long time this man had not worn clothes or lived in a house, but had lived in the tombs. When he saw Jesus, he cried out and fell at his feet, shouting at the top of his voice, "What do you want with me, Jesus, Son of the Most High God? I beg you, don't torture me!"

For Jesus had commanded the impure spirit to come out of the man. Many times it had seized him, and though he was chained hand and foot and kept under guard, he had broken his chains and had been driven by the demon into solitary places.

Jesus asked him, "What is your name?" "Legion," he replied, because many demons had gone into him. And they begged Jesus repeatedly not to order them to go into the abyss. A large herd of pigs was feeding there on the hillside. The demons begged Jesus to let them go into the pigs, and he gave them permission. When the demons came out of the man, they went into the pigs, and the herd rushed down the steep bank into the lake and was drowned. When those tending the pigs saw what had happened, they ran off and reported this in the town and countryside, and the people went out to see what had happened. When they came to Jesus, they found the man from whom the demons had gone out, sitting at Jesus' feet, dressed and in his right mind; and they were afraid.

Those who had seen it told the people how the demon-possessed man had been cured. Then all the people of the region of the Gerasenes asked Jesus to leave them because they were overcome with fear. So he got into the boat and left. The man from whom the demons had gone out begged to go with him, but Jesus sent him away, saying, "Return home and tell how much God has done for you." So the man went away and told all over town how much Jesus had done for him.

Application Questions

? How would you react if a naked man came running towards you and shouting?

_____

? How did Jesus react?

_____

? What does this teach you about the nature of Jesus?

? What kind of interactions have you had with homeless people?

? What do you need restoration from?

? After Jesus restored the man, what does he tell him to do?

? When Jesus restores us from bondage, what should we do?

Key Concepts

Jesus has the power to restore you from anything that possesses you. He, alone, has the power to restore you from the bondage of food. Once you are restored, you should be telling others about the power and work of Jesus

Weekly Challenges

A. Make *THREE NEW* Weekly Commitments:

① _____

② _____

③ _____

B. Meet With Your Accountability Partner at least once this week.

C. Weigh yourself on Monday morning, and record your weight. Weigh yourself again on Sunday evening, and record the weight.

_____   _____
Monday Morning Weight   Sunday Night Weight

C. Use a Journal to record every time you eat when you're not truly hungry. See if you can find a pattern/ trigger.

D. Memory Verse:
Proverbs 25:28
Like a city whose walls are broken through is a person who lacks self-control.

Hunger Scale Accountability Chart

0	1	2	3	4	5
Hungry Hungry Hippo	Stomach Growling	Hungry	Not Hungry	Satisfied	Stuffed

	NOTE: Try and avoid the snack whenever possible.	Meal 1	Meal 2	Snack
Sample	Level When You Started Eating	1.3	2.0	
	Level When You Finished Eating	3.2	4.2	
DAY 1	Level When You Started Eating			
	Level When You Finished Eating			
DAY 2	Level When You Started Eating			
	Level When You Finished Eating			
DAY 3	Level When You Started Eating			
	Level When You Finished Eating			
DAY 4	Level When You Started Eating			
	Level When You Finished Eating			
DAY 5	Level When You Started Eating			
	Level When You Finished Eating			
DAY 6	Level When You Started Eating			
	Level When You Finished Eating			
DAY 7	Level When You Started Eating			
	Level When You Finished Eating			

End of Week Accountability Questions

1. Did you eat when you were at 0, 1, or 2 on the hunger scale and ask God for strength to wait till you reached one of those levels before eating? ○ Yes   ○ No
2. Once you reached the point when your stomach was growling or was empty, did you eat foods that you love and that are 4 or 5 stars? ○ Yes   ○ No
3. Did you stop before you were full at a level 4, and did you eat slowly in a non-stressful environment and savor your food? ○ Yes   ○ No
4. Did you eat real foods without chemicals and limit sugar consumption? (Remember: None of the thin eaters counted carbs or removed sugar when they wanted to lose weight, but they did consciously limit sugar) ○ Yes   ○ No
5. Did you eat when a stressful situation came up this week? ○ Yes   ○ No
6. Did you eat for any other reason than true hunger this week? ○ Yes   ○ No
7. Did you ever feel tired/sluggish after eating? ○ Yes   ○ No

Friend Accountability Chart

Name	Email	Social Media Info	# of Times Contacted	Method Used

Weekly Accountability Chart

	Yes	No
Did you experience any temptation breakthroughs (like the cake story on page 43) this week or any time God provided a way out for you, so you didn't eat when you weren't hungry?		
Did you spend less time thinking about food?		
Are you starting to understand that you can eat what you want within your red, yellow, green light foods? (See page 80)		
Are you starting to eat ½ to ⅔ what you used to?		
Are you slowing down when you eat?		
Did you pick a fasting window and stick to it? (See page 30)		
Did you memorize any Bible verses to help you?		

Your Success Stories

It's important to celebrate your accomplishments! In *Fasting to Freedom*, I talk about enslaving sins. They cannot be fixed overnight. They take time to overcome. I cannot eat slowly; I've gotten better, but I'm not perfect. So I celebrate the other things I've learned to do well.

Rate how well you did (1-10) with these concepts over the past week:

Success	Rating
I tried an extended 24 hour fast	
I fasted longer than last week	
I put my fork down between each bite	
I cut my food portion in ½ or ⅓	
I did a quiet time every morning/night *Joshua 1:8* *Keep this Book of the Law always on your lips; meditate on it day and night, so that you may be careful to do everything written in it. Then you will be prosperous and successful.*	
I found an accountability partner to do an extended fast with me	
I ate the best foods on my plate first	
If I overate, I waited to do a 24-hour fast and got all the way to empty and hungry before eating again	
I ate more slowly than the day before	
I chose nutrient-dense foods	
I cut back on sugar	
I tried to eat more slowly	
I ate real foods without a lot of chemicals	

Success	Rating
I took smaller portions to begin with	
I asked the Holy Spirit to help me avoid eating when not hungry and to avoid false hunger	
I never ate beyond level 4 on the hunger scale	
I stopped eating at a 3.8 knowing that within 20 minutes I would be at a level 4	
I ate what I was craving instead of diet foods	
I only ate 1 or 2 meals a day and didn't fast	
I ate at a level 0, 1, or 2	
I prayed for discernment before I ate	
I didn't drink sweet beverages like sweet tea or sugary drinks or use gum/mints between mealtimes.	
I drank no calories drinks	

Weekly Prayer:

"God I want to get into a right relationship with food and only eat when I'm truly hungry and stop when I'm full. I never want to yo-yo diet again. Please let the Holy Spirit intervene whenever I'm about to overeat, and help so I **don't** overeat. Help me to slow down and savor my food and help me to fall in love with You, not food; let You be my fiancé and my go to, not the food." (See explanation on page 82)

Make your own prayer based on what you want to work on for the week:

_____

_____

_____

Bonus Session 1: Discernment vs. Deprivation

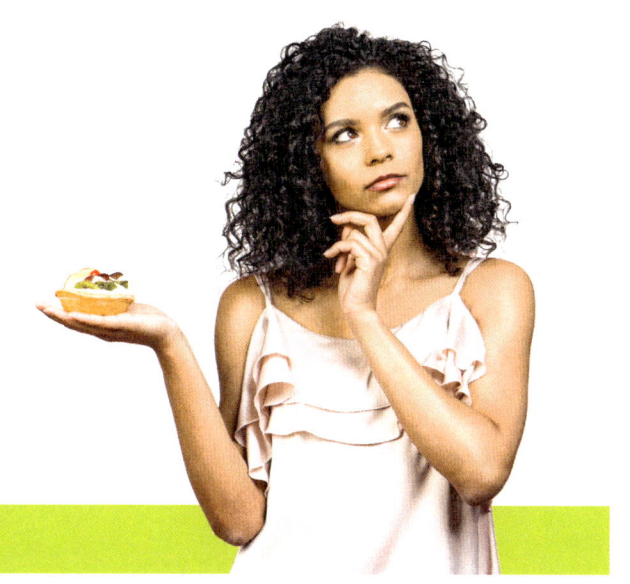

Weekly Ice Breaker

Peaks and Pits — Think about the past week. What were your Peaks and your Pits?

These can be food/eating-related but don't have to be. Your Peaks should be things that brought you joy, made you feel happy, made you smile, made you feel energized or excited — things you enjoyed and would enjoy doing again. Your Pits should be things that drained your energy, made you upset or angry, made you sad, made you frustrated, or gave you a headache — things you wish you didn't have to repeat again.

Now, write them in the spaces below:

Peaks	Pits

Weekly Game

I went to the Supermarket: One person starts with the phrase: "I went to the supermarket and I bought…" It can be whatever you like. For example, the first person says, "An avocado", the next person will say, "I went to the supermarket with (add in the first person's name) and I bought an avocado… and a chocolate bar."

Each person adds their own item to the end of the list but must remembers everyone else's names and items who went before them. Can't remember an item? You're out!

Psalm 81:10
I am the LORD your God, who brought you up out of Egypt.
Open wide your mouth and I will fill it.

Key Concepts

The problem with diets is that they force us to focus more on food. They create a big greed problem because instead of addressing the problem of overeating, they encourage us to have larger amounts of food. They justify it by labeling some foods as "good" and others as "bad." We need to fix the root of the problem, not the food choice. It's all about self-control. Think discernment, not deprivation. Even if you're eating healthfully, you can still overeat and consume too many calories. You can still gorge on "good" foods. Tell yourself, "I am not depriving myself of anything. If there is anything I want to eat, I may eat it. I am going to make wise choices and I'm not going to eat everything at once. If I want half of a donut, I can have half of a donut. I'm not going to be afraid of eating certain things."

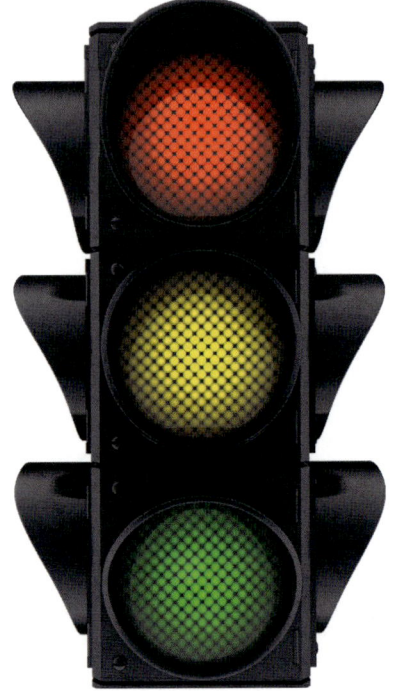

Red Light, Yellow Light, Green Light Foods:

You can eat whatever you want, but you must create a list for yourself that asks, "How do I feel when I eat these foods?" No one is ever telling you that you cannot eat something. If you don't have any issues and are healthy, then you should eat whatever you want, and you should not deprive yourself. Now, if you are sick like me, then you have to be discerning about which foods you put in your body because if you eat certain foods you will feel so terrible that it's just not worth it. The key is to make substitutions. You have to discern for yourself which foods are your own red lights, yellow lights, or green lights.

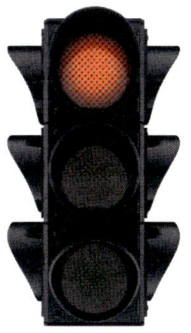
Red Light Foods
Foods that your body cannot handle, and you must avoid. For me this is gluten, legumes, and most dairy.

Yellow Light Foods
Foods that your body feels okay eating occasionally, but you must limit them. For me this is corn, white rice, and goat's milk.

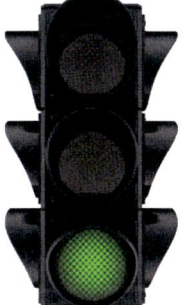
Green Light Foods
Foods that your body feels good eating and you do not need to limit. For me this is fruits, lean meats, and non-starchy vegetables.

Everyone has a different opinion about what real food is, some people think real food is whole milk, cream, fresh farm eggs, garden vegetables, whole cuts of steak, and hamburger, fruits, cheeses, etc. But if you look at a typical grocery store 80% of the food at the grocery store isn't whole foods anymore. It's all highly processed foods. An entire aisle is for cereal, crackers, sodas, chips. Only the outer perimeters have fruits, vegetables meats, and cheeses. Everything in the middle is a processed food. The only things most people agree are really good for you are vegetables. The problem with our food is that even things like yogurt are processed.

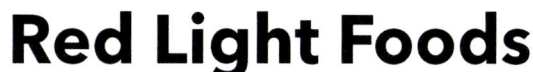

The Doughnut Story

One time I had an assistant who had these mini-donuts sitting on her desk for 3-days, and for 3-days they tempted me. So one day, when she called out sick, I took them off her desk and devoured them! I felt so guilty about stealing the donuts that I immediately went to the store and replaced them for her. But I also felt anger at myself for having so little self-control that I couldn't even resist some processed, store-bought mini-donuts. If I wanted a donut, I should have gotten a better quality or gluten-free one instead of giving into temptation and eating processed junk food!

Application Questions

? Why is depriving yourself a bad idea?

___

? Are there some foods that you eat even though they make you feel bad?

___

? What are some substitutions you could make in your diet so that you can eat what you're craving but still feel your best?

___

? What foods do you think are healthful but are actually not?

___

? Watch the video on chantelrayway.com/biblestudy called, "Do You Diet?" Did the thin eaters diet? Why or why not??

Food As Your Fiancé

If you think about when someone has a fiancé, it's usually the happiest time in their relationship. They're both excited; they seem to sparkle when they're together. A person's fiancé is their source of happiness, comfort, and excitement. We can have the same emotions with food. As soon as you see food, your pulse goes up, you get excited. Food becomes your go-to for emotional support.

False hunger: Food is your false friend, false comfort, false encouragement, false support, false shoulder to cry on.

We need God to be our fiancé, our shoulder to cry on, our bride-groom, the one to go to for comfort and security. I know that when I indulge in food, it's five minutes. Ask yourself: Is it worth it to trade a lifetime of thinness, body confidence and health for five minutes of indulgence?

Tell yourself:

I'M NOT GOING TO CHOOSE FIVE MINUTES OF GLUTTONY OVER A LIFETIME OF BEING THIN. BEING THIN FAR OUTWEIGHS OVEREATING. I'M ALSO SINNING BY OVEREATING.

The Devils's Big Fat Lies

James 4:7-10
Submit yourselves, then, to God. Resist the devil, and he will flee from you. Come near to God and he will come near to you. Wash your hands, you sinners, and purify your hearts, you double-minded. Grieve, mourn and wail. Change your laughter to mourning and your joy to gloom. Humble yourselves before the Lord, and he will lift you up.

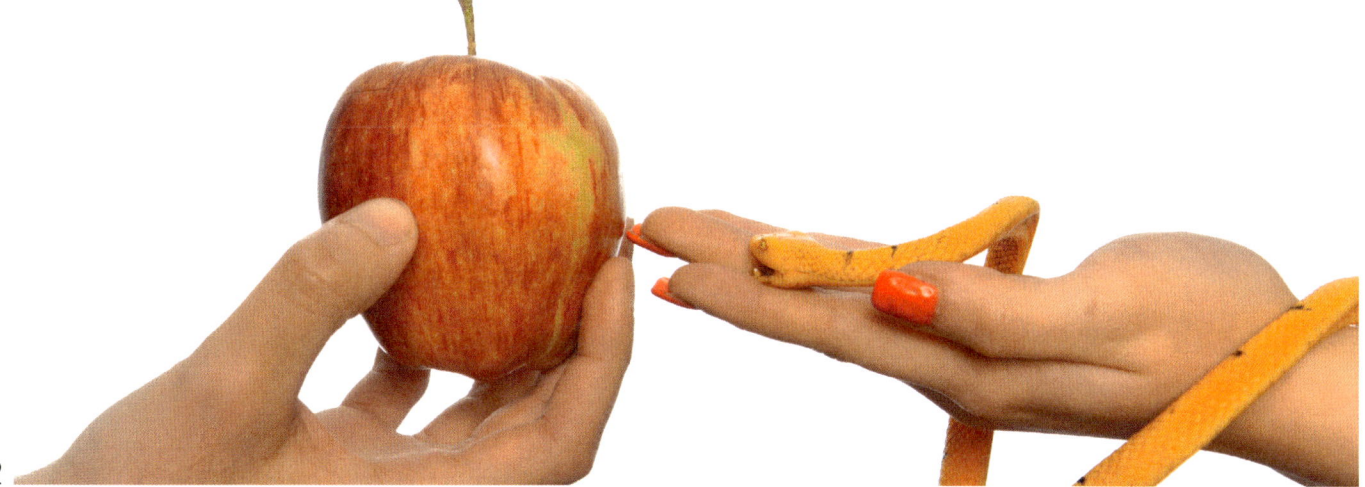

These are the types of the lies I've heard over and over:

- I have a low metabolism, so I can't eat whatever I want like other girls.
- It's my birthday; I definitely need at least two pieces of cake.
- It's Thanksgiving; everyone overeats on Thanksgiving, so it's okay if I do.
- I have four kids and work full-time; I don't have time to spend with God or to memorize Bible verses.
- It's the Christmas party at Ruth's Chris; I can't let this good of food go to waste.

Application Questions

? On which holiday do you allow yourself to overeat?

_____

_____

? Has the devil ever used these lies or similar ones on you? Which ones?

_____

_____

? Are there any lies you've overcome? What were they?

_____

_____

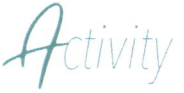

Break into partners and read these lies that the devil tries to tell you, and the truths that counter them, then write down some other lies the devil puts in your life and the truths.

Lies	Truths
You already waited till 11am, and your stomach hasn't growled, so you might as well just eat.	No, I will wait until my stomach is fully empty and growls.
You're at work and your stomach isn't growling yet, but you won't have a break until later, so you better eat now.	It's not the end of world if I feel hungry and eat a little later. I can eat at my next break, and my body will burn fat when my stomach growls.
You've been in bondage to food for 30 years; it won't change. You will always be fat, so you should just enjoy this.	Enslaving sins are not overcome overnight; even if I've been struggling for years, I can overcome them with the help of the Holy Spirit.
You're celebrating your grandmother's birthday at Ruth's Chris; You won't be back here for a long time, so you might as well overeat just this once.	I must break the habit of overeating no matter where I am. I can save my leftovers and bring them home to enjoy again.
You don't feel well, but food will make you feel better.	If I'm physically hungry, then I should eat, but I'm not, then eating will only make me feel worse.
You're going to be drinking a lot tonight; you better eat a big meal, so you don't get drunk.	The best thing I can do when I'm drinking alcohol is also drink plenty of water!
You're satisfied and don't want dessert, but it's your friend's birthday, so you better eat a piece of cake to make her happy.	I can have just a couple bites of the cake; I don't have to eat a whole slice, and a real friend is just glad I'm there celebrating and doesn't care whether I'm eating.
Your work out at the gym today was really hard. You deserve to indulge in a whole pan of brownies.	There's never an excuse to sin and overeat, no matter how hard I worked out. Why would I want to overeat and ruin it after working so hard at the gym to look and feel good?
You had a terrible day at work; comfort food will help.	Overeating will only make me feel physically and emotionally worse.

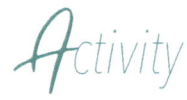

Use this space below to write your own answers.

Lies	Truths

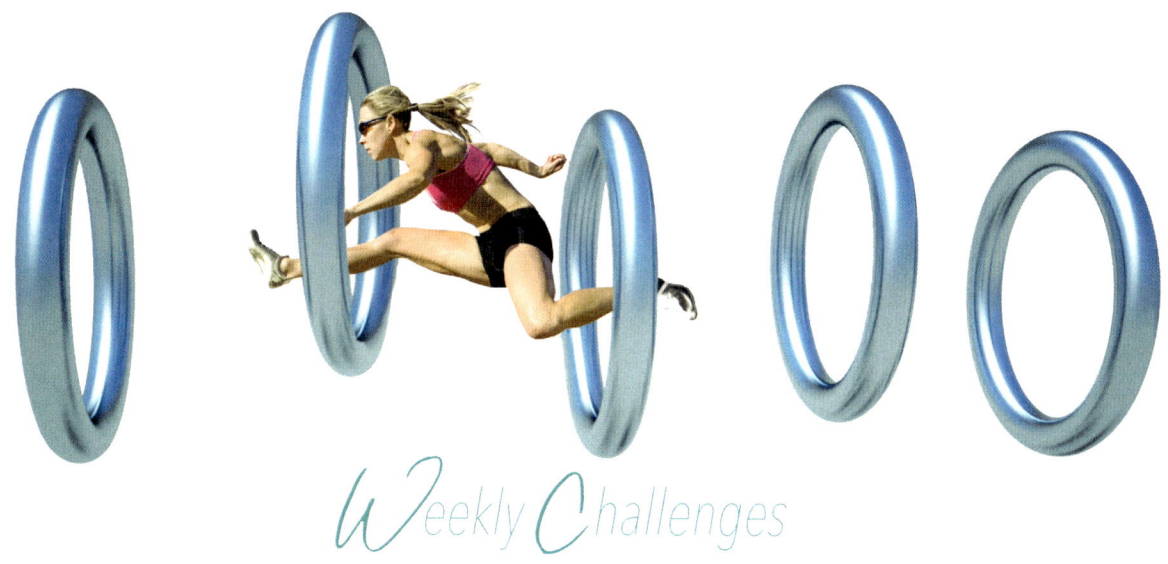

Weekly Challenges

A. Make *THREE NEW* Weekly Commitments:

❶ _____

_____

❷ _____

_____

❸ _____

_____

B. Meet With Your Accountability Partner at least once this week.

C. Weigh yourself on Monday morning, and record your weight. Weigh yourself again on Sunday evening, and record the weight.

_____   _____
Monday Morning Weight   Sunday Night Weight

C. Use a Journal to record every time you eat when you're not truly hungry. See if you can find a pattern/ trigger.

D. Memory Verse:

Proverbs 25:28
Like a city whose walls are broken through is a person who lacks self-control.

Hunger Scale Accountability Chart

0 Hungry Hungry Hippo
1 Stomach Growling
2 Hungry
3 Not Hungry
4 Satisfied
5 Stuffed

	NOTE: Try and avoid the snack whenever possible.	Meal 1	Meal 2	Snack
Sample	Level When You Started Eating	1.3	2.0	
	Level When You Finished Eating	3.2	4.2	
DAY 1	Level When You Started Eating			
	Level When You Finished Eating			
DAY 2	Level When You Started Eating			
	Level When You Finished Eating			
DAY 3	Level When You Started Eating			
	Level When You Finished Eating			
DAY 4	Level When You Started Eating			
	Level When You Finished Eating			
DAY 5	Level When You Started Eating			
	Level When You Finished Eating			
DAY 6	Level When You Started Eating			
	Level When You Finished Eating			
DAY 7	Level When You Started Eating			
	Level When You Finished Eating			

End of Week Accountability Questions

1. Did you eat when you were at 0, 1, or 2 on the hunger scale and ask God for strength to wait till you reached one of those levels before eating? ○ Yes   ○ No
2. Once you reached the point when your stomach was growling or was empty, did you eat foods that you love and that are 4 or 5 stars? ○ Yes   ○ No
3. Did you stop before you were full at a level 4, and did you eat slowly in a non-stressful environment and savor your food? ○ Yes   ○ No
4. Did you eat real foods without chemicals and limit sugar consumption? (Remember: None of the thin eaters counted carbs or removed sugar when they wanted to lose weight, but they did consciously limit sugar) ○ Yes   ○ No
5. Did you eat when a stressful situation came up this week? ○ Yes   ○ No
6. Did you eat for any other reason than true hunger this week? ○ Yes   ○ No
7. Did you ever feel tired/sluggish after eating? ○ Yes   ○ No

Friend Accountability Chart

Name	Email	Social Media Info	# of Times Contacted	Method Used

Weekly Accountability Chart

	Yes	No
Did you experience any temptation breakthroughs (like the cake story on page 43) this week or any time God provided a way out for you, so you didn't eat when you weren't hungry?		
Did you spend less time thinking about food?		
Are you starting to understand that you can eat what you want within your red, yellow, green light foods? (See page 80)		
Are you starting to eat ½ to ⅔ what you used to?		
Are you slowing down when you eat?		
Did you pick a fasting window and stick to it? (See page 30)		
Did you memorize any Bible verses to help you?		

Your Success Stories

It's important to celebrate your accomplishments! In *Fasting to Freedom*, I talk about enslaving sins. They cannot be fixed overnight. They take time to overcome. I cannot eat slowly; I've gotten better, but I'm not perfect. So I celebrate the other things I've learned to do well.

Rate how well you did (1-10) with these concepts over the past week:

Success	Rating
I tried an extended 24 hour fast	
I fasted longer than last week	
I put my fork down between each bite	
I cut my food portion in ½ or ⅓	
I did a quiet time every morning/night *Joshua 1:8* *Keep this Book of the Law always on your lips; meditate on it day and night, so that you may be careful to do everything written in it. Then you will be prosperous and successful.*	
I found an accountability partner to do an extended fast with me	
I ate the best foods on my plate first	
If I overate, I waited to do a 24-hour fast and got all the way to empty and hungry before eating again	
I ate more slowly than the day before	
I chose nutrient-dense foods	
I cut back on sugar	
I tried to eat more slowly	
I ate real foods without a lot of chemicals	

Success	Rating
I took smaller portions to begin with	
I asked the Holy Spirit to help me avoid eating when not hungry and to avoid false hunger	
I never ate beyond level 4 on the hunger scale	
I stopped eating at a 3.8 knowing that within 20 minutes I would be at a level 4	
I ate what I was craving instead of diet foods	
I only ate 1 or 2 meals a day and didn't fast	
I ate at a level 0, 1, or 2	
I prayed for discernment before I ate	
I didn't drink sweet beverages like sweet tea or sugary drinks or use gum/mints between mealtimes.	
I drank no calories drinks	

Weekly Prayer:

"God I want to get into a right relationship with food and only eat when I'm truly hungry and stop when I'm full. I never want to yo-yo diet again. Please let the Holy Spirit intervene whenever I'm about to overeat, and help so I **don't** overeat. Help me to slow down and savor my food and help me to fall in love with You, not food; let You be my fiancé and my go to, not the food." (See explanation on page 82)

Make your own prayer based on what you want to work on for the week:

_____

_____

_____

_____

Bonus Session 2: Take Care of Yourself First

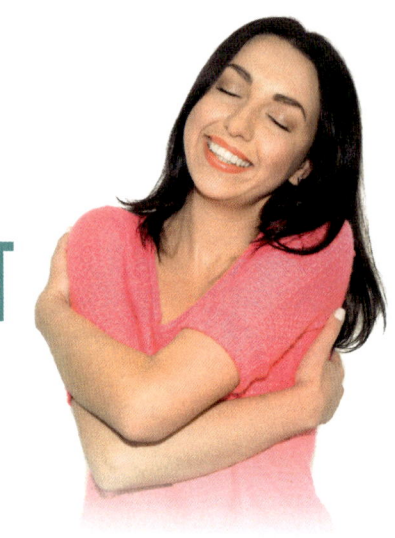

Weekly Ice Breaker

Peaks and Pits – Think about the past week. What were your Peaks and your Pits?

These can be food/eating-related but don't have to be. Your Peaks should be things that brought you joy, made you feel happy, made you smile, made you feel energized or excited – things you enjoyed and would enjoy doing again. Your Pits should be things that drained your energy, made you upset or angry, made you sad, made you frustrated, or gave you a headache – things you wish you didn't have to repeat again.

Now, write them in the spaces below:

Peaks	Pits

Weekly Game

Lucky Penny: Everyone grab a coin from your purse and look at the date. Now go around and one-by-one tell something interesting that happened to you in the year that's on your coin.

Mark 6:31-32
Then, because so many people were coming and going that they did not even have a chance to eat, he said to them, "Come with me by yourselves to a quiet place and get some rest." So they went away by themselves in a boat to a solitary place.

3 John 1:2
Dear friend, I pray that you may enjoy good health and that all may go well with you, even as your soul is getting along well.

Key Concepts

Everyone knows that when you're on a plane, the flight attendants instruct you, in case of an emergency, to put on your own oxygen mask before assisting your children with theirs, and this might seem selfish, but if we pass out, we can't help others stay alive. Most Christians think they must only do for others and practice selflessness, in fact most Bible verses focus on teaching us to do for others because, as humans, we are naturally self-centered. However, as women and mothers, there are many times when we get so caught up in making sure our families are cared for, that we forget to care for ourselves.

You Cannot Pour From an Empty Cup

If we do not make the time to care for ourselves, eventually our bodies will give out, and we will not be able to care for others. Remember 1 Corinthians 3:16-17 *Don't you know that you yourselves are God's temple and that God's Spirit dwells in your midst?*

Your body is God's temple, and you are called to care for it.
Not caring for God's temple is a sin.

Application Questions

? When was the last time you took the time to care for yourself?

___

? What's something you could do for yourself in the next week?

___

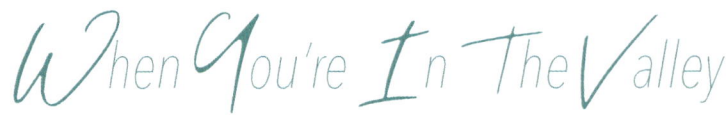
When You're In The Valley

Ezekiel 37: 1-14

The hand of the LORD was on me, and he brought me out by the Spirit of the LORD and set me in the middle of a valley; it was full of bones. He led me back and forth among them, and I saw a great many bones on the floor of the valley, bones that were very dry. He asked me, "Son of man, can these bones live?"

I said, "Sovereign LORD, you alone know."

Then he said to me, "Prophesy to these bones and say to them, 'Dry bones, hear the word of the LORD! This is what the Sovereign LORD says to these bones: I will make breath[a] enter you, and you will come to life. I will attach tendons to you and make flesh come upon you and cover you with skin; I will put breath in you, and you will come to life. Then you will know that I am the LORD.'"

So I prophesied as I was commanded. And as I was prophesying, there was a noise, a rattling sound, and the bones came together, bone to bone. I looked, and tendons and flesh appeared on them and skin covered them, but there was no breath in them.

Then he said to me, "Prophesy to the breath; prophesy, son of man, and say to it, 'This is what the Sovereign LORD says: Come, breath, from the four winds and breathe into these slain, that they may live.'" So I prophesied as he commanded me, and breath entered them; they came to life and stood up on their feet—a vast army.

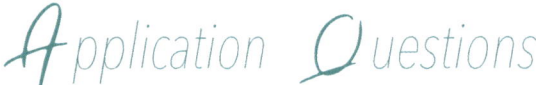
Application Questions

? What is the valley?

_____

? What valley are you going through right now?

_____

? Why does God take us through valleys?

_____

Key Concepts

The valley is a place of challenge, it is the gym of the Holy Spirit; it hurts but it's good for you. God is always with you in the valley – "...the hand of God was on me." Your struggle with food is a valley. There's no fruit in the mountaintop; there's only fruit in the valley. Growth and strength come from the valley.

God is not going to give you a life where he is unnecessary; your challenges serve his purpose. You have to learn to give God your not enough/your challenges because God can bless it until you have more than enough. You must speak to whatever you're facing. When you speak God's word, things will happen. The Holy Spirit will breathe on your life: "...Breath entered them; they came to life..."

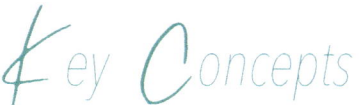

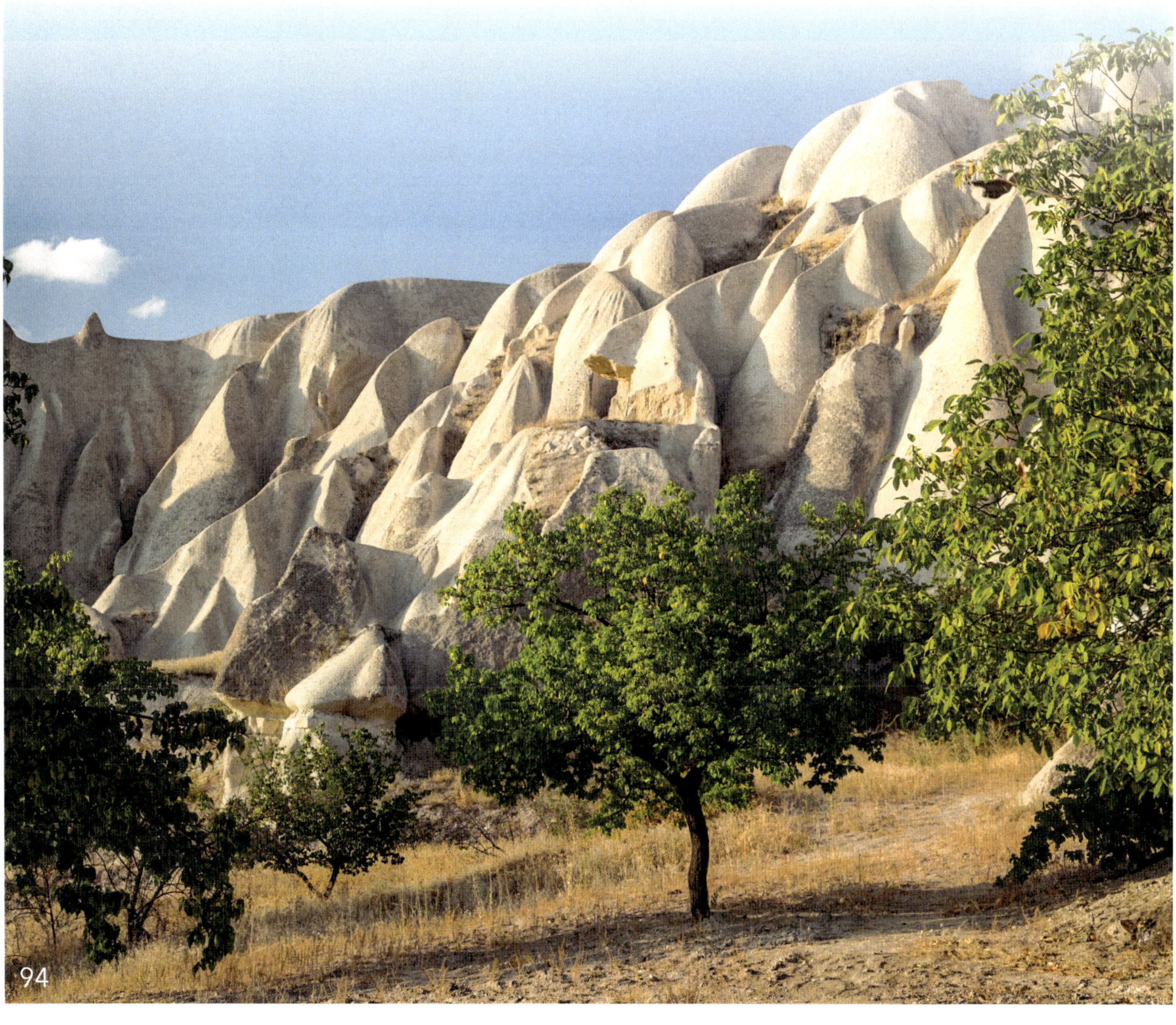

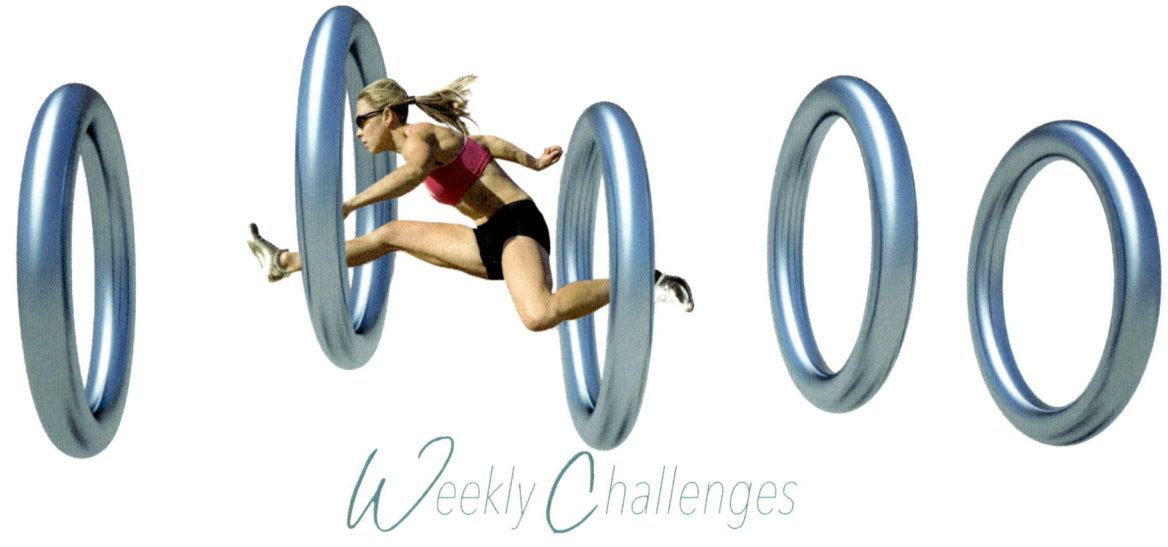

Weekly Challenges

A. **Do at least one thing to care for yourself this week.**

B. **Make *THREE NEW* Weekly Commitments:**

❶ _____

_____

❷ _____

_____

❸ _____

_____

C. **Meet With Your Accountability Partner** at least once this week.

D. **Weigh yourself** on Monday morning, and record your weight. Weigh yourself again on Sunday evening, and record the weight.

_____   _____
Monday Morning Weight   Sunday Night Weight

E. **Use a Journal** to record every time you eat when you're not truly hungry. See if you can find a pattern/ trigger.

F. **Memory Verse:**

1 Peter 3:4
Rather, it should be that of your inner self, the unfading beauty of a gentle and quiet spirit, which is of great worth in God's sight.

Hunger Scale Accountability Chart

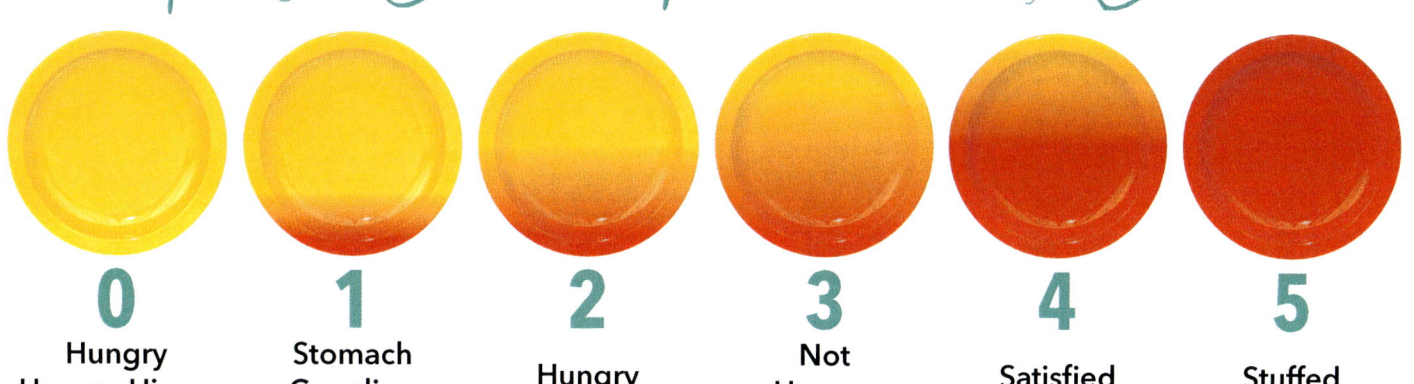

0	1	2	3	4	5
Hungry Hungry Hippo	Stomach Growling	Hungry	Not Hungry	Satisfied	Stuffed

	NOTE: Try and avoid the snack whenever possible.	Meal 1	Meal 2	Snack
Sample	Level When You Started Eating	1.3	2.0	
	Level When You Finished Eating	3.2	4.2	
DAY 1	Level When You Started Eating			
	Level When You Finished Eating			
DAY 2	Level When You Started Eating			
	Level When You Finished Eating			
DAY 3	Level When You Started Eating			
	Level When You Finished Eating			
DAY 4	Level When You Started Eating			
	Level When You Finished Eating			
DAY 5	Level When You Started Eating			
	Level When You Finished Eating			
DAY 6	Level When You Started Eating			
	Level When You Finished Eating			
DAY 7	Level When You Started Eating			
	Level When You Finished Eating			

End of Week Accountability Questions

1. Did you eat when you were at 0, 1, or 2 on the hunger scale and ask God for strength to wait till you reached one of those levels before eating? ○ Yes   ○ No
2. Once you reached the point when your stomach was growling or was empty, did you eat foods that you love and that are 4 or 5 stars? ○ Yes   ○ No
3. Did you stop before you were full at a level 4, and did you eat slowly in a non-stressful environment and savor your food? ○ Yes   ○ No
4. Did you eat real foods without chemicals and limit sugar consumption? (Remember: None of the thin eaters counted carbs or removed sugar when they wanted to lose weight, but they did consciously limit sugar) ○ Yes   ○ No
5. Did you eat when a stressful situation came up this week? ○ Yes   ○ No
6. Did you eat for any other reason than true hunger this week? ○ Yes   ○ No
7. Did you ever feel tired/sluggish after eating? ○ Yes   ○ No

Friend Accountability Chart

Name	Email	Social Media Info	# of Times Contacted	Method Used

Weekly Accountability Chart

	Yes	No
Did you experience any temptation breakthroughs (like the cake story on page 43) this week or any time God provided a way out for you, so you didn't eat when you weren't hungry?		
Did you spend less time thinking about food?		
Are you starting to understand that you can eat what you want within your red, yellow, green light foods? (See page 80)		
Are you starting to eat ½ to ⅔ what you used to?		
Are you slowing down when you eat?		
Did you pick a fasting window and stick to it? (See page 30)		
Did you memorize any Bible verses to help you?		

Your Success Stories

It's important to celebrate your accomplishments! In *Fasting to Freedom*, I talk about enslaving sins. They cannot be fixed overnight. They take time to overcome. I cannot eat slowly; I've gotten better, but I'm not perfect. So I celebrate the other things I've learned to do well.

Rate how well you did (1-10) with these concepts over the past week:

Success	Rating
I tried an extended 24 hour fast	
I fasted longer than last week	
I put my fork down between each bite	
I cut my food portion in ½ or ⅓	
I did a quiet time every morning/night *Joshua 1:8* *Keep this Book of the Law always on your lips; meditate on it day and night, so that you may be careful to do everything written in it. Then you will be prosperous and successful.*	
I found an accountability partner to do an extended fast with me	
I ate the best foods on my plate first	
If I overate, I waited to do a 24-hour fast and got all the way to empty and hungry before eating again	
I ate more slowly than the day before	
I chose nutrient-dense foods	
I cut back on sugar	
I tried to eat more slowly	
I ate real foods without a lot of chemicals	

Success	Rating
I took smaller portions to begin with	
I asked the Holy Spirit to help me avoid eating when not hungry and to avoid false hunger	
I never ate beyond level 4 on the hunger scale	
I stopped eating at a 3.8 knowing that within 20 minutes I would be at a level 4	
I ate what I was craving instead of diet foods	
I only ate 1 or 2 meals a day and didn't fast	
I ate at a level 0, 1, or 2	
I prayed for discernment before I ate	
I didn't drink sweet beverages like sweet tea or sugary drinks or use gum/mints between mealtimes.	
I drank no calories drinks	

Weekly Prayer:

"God I want to get into a right relationship with food and only eat when I'm truly hungry and stop when I'm full. I never want to yo-yo diet again. Please let the Holy Spirit intervene whenever I'm about to overeat, and help so I **don't** overeat. Help me to slow down and savor my food and help me to fall in love with You, not food; let You be my fiancé and my go to, not the food." (See explanation on page 82)

Make your own prayer based on what you want to work on for the week:

_____

_____

_____

_____

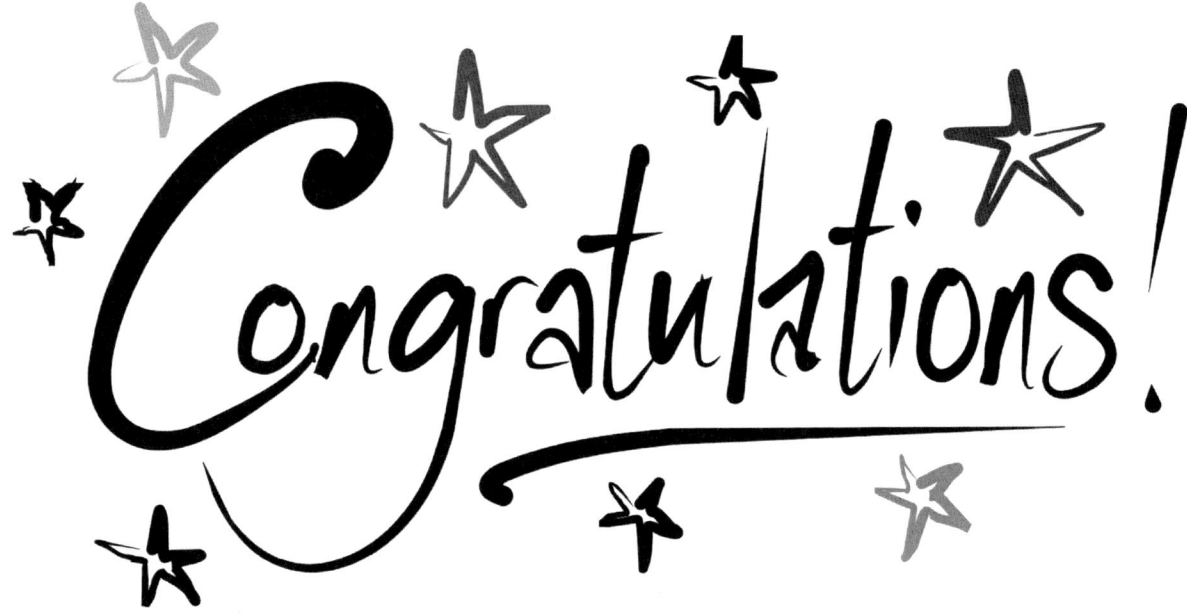

Now that you have spent six weeks discovering how to use the Holy Spirit & God's Word to escape temptation and avoid sinning when you eat, your adventure as a thin person has just begun! Don't forget the lessons of this workbook. Return to them if you ever struggle, and share the concepts with others. Remember, you are never alone, and are not expected to break old habits by yourself—the Holy Spirit is always available, as is the Word of God. It is sharper than any two-edged sword, and is the best weapon against the enemy. (Not to mention a sharp sword cuts through a beautiful slice of cake as thinly as you actually want.)

Enjoy your food; enjoy your life!

Chantel Ray

Made in the USA
Coppell, TX
27 May 2022

78209510R00064